Disclaimer

The author has made every attempt to be as accurate and complete as possible in the creation of this publication, however he / she does not warrant or represent at any time that the contents within are accurate due to the rapidly changing nature of the Internet. The author assumes no responsibility for errors, omissions, or contrary interpretation of the subject matter herein. Any perceived slights of specific persons, peoples, or organizations other published materials are unintentional and used solely for educational purposes only.

This information is not intended for use as a source of legal, business, accounting or financial and investment advice. All readers are advised to seek services of competent professionals in legal, business, accounting, investment and finance field. No representation is made or implied that the reader will do as well from using the suggested techniques, strategies, methods, systems, or ideas; rather it is presented for news value only.

The author does not assume any responsibility or liability whatsoever for what you choose to do with this information. Use your own judgment. Under no circumstances will the product creator, programmer or any of the distributors of this product, or any distributors, be liable to any party for any direct, indirect, punitive, special, incidental, or other consequential damages arising directly or indirectly from the use of this product. This product is provided "as is" and without warranties.

Consult appropriate professionals before starting a business.

Any perceived remark, or similarities of trademark, comment or use of organizations, people mentioned and any resemblance to characters living, dead or otherwise, real or fictitious does not mean that they support this content in any way.

There are no guarantees of income made, traffic delivered or other promises of any kind. Readers are cautioned to reply on their own judgment about their individual circumstances to act accordingly. By reading any document, the reader agrees that under no circumstances is the author responsible for any losses, direct or indirect, that are incurred as a result of use of the information contained within this document, including - but not limited to errors, omissions, or inaccuracies.

Copyright@ Selena Harris 2023

Table of Contents

Introduction

Chapter 1- Initiation to Healthy Eating for Growing Teenagers

1.1 What is healthy food?

1.2 How to introduce healthy eating habits for teenagers?

1.3 Why should teens eat healthy food?

Chapter 2- Identifying Nutritional Needs for Teenagers

2.1 Instigate what the nutritional needs are in teenagers.

2.2 Find out why nutrition is required for teenagers.

2.3 What is the role of parents in ensuring adequate nutrition?

Chapter 3- Understanding Macronutrients and Their Benefits

3.1 Macronutrients: What Are They?

3.2 What are the benefits of macronutrients?

3.3 Combinations and timings of macronutrients.

3.4 Why is it essential to have macronutrients for teenagers?

Chapter 4- Planning Healthy Meals for Teenagers

4.1 What is the definition of a healthy meal?

4.2 Learn the benefits of eating healthy.

4.3 Planning healthy meals for teenagers.

4.4 Encouraging healthy eating habits for teens.

Chapter 5- Shopping for Healthy Foods

5.1 Learn a few tips for shopping for healthy foods.

5.2 Comparison between the benefits of buying local and organic?

5.3 Pick up some tips for eating healthy on a budget.

Chapter 6- Making Healthy Choices at Home

6.1 Determine meal planning and preparation.

6.2 Pursue limiting processed foods.

6.3 Why is staying hydrated equally important as healthy eating?

Chapter 7- Strategies for Eating Healthy While Out

7.1 Learn a few healthy eating-out options.

7.2 How to have a balanced food platter?

7.3 Re-think about your drinks.

Chapter 8- Creating an Exercise Plan

8.1 What are the benefits of exercising regularly?

8.2 How to implement an exercise routine?

Chapter 9- Staying Motivated to Adopt a Healthy Lifestyle

9.1 Get trained on setting realistic goals.

9.2 Finding the right support system.

9.3 Go ahead with celebrating your achievements.

Chapter 10- Case Study on Healthy Eating for Growing Teenagers.

Conclusion

Introduction

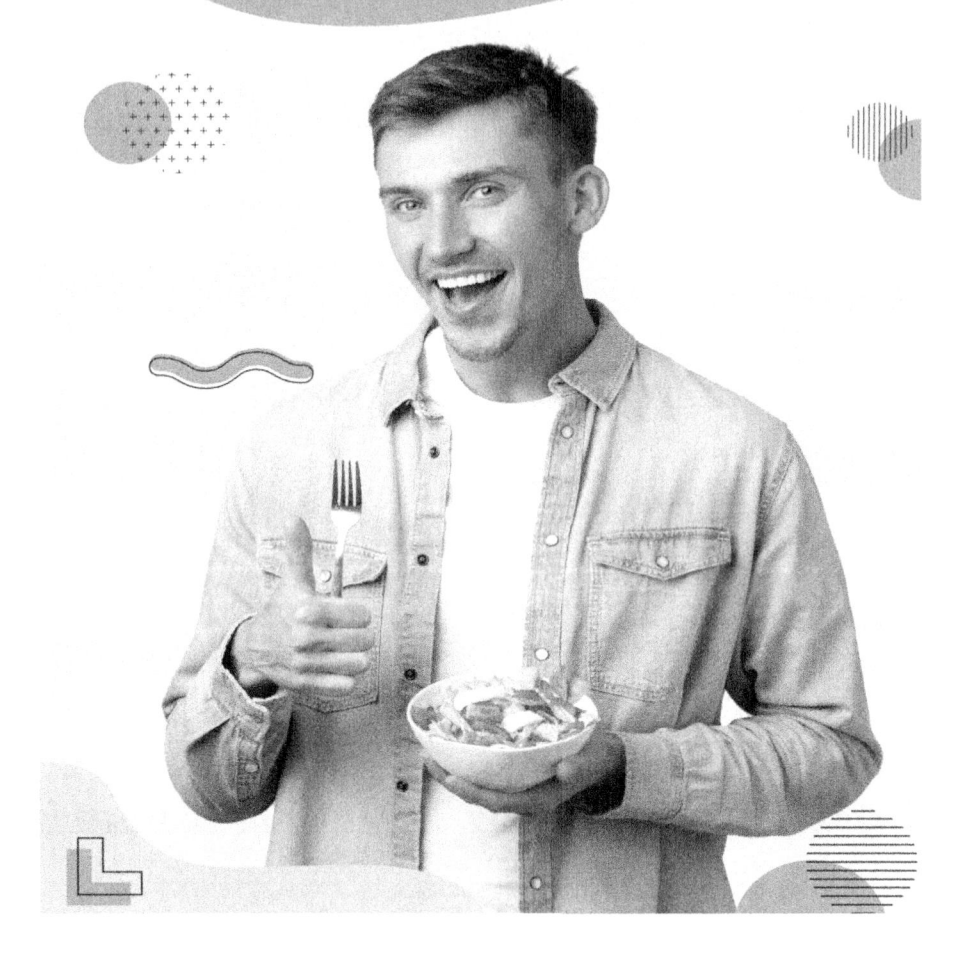

Teenagers must remember that their bodies are rapidly developing as they enter their teenage years. That is why it is so important for teens to eat a healthy, balanced diet.

Unfortunately, many teenagers do not take healthy eating seriously and, as a result, can suffer from various drawbacks.

Healthy eating is essential for teenage growth and development. Eating a balanced diet helps teenagers stay healthy, grow properly, and maintain a healthy weight.

This training guide will provide an overview of healthy eating for growing teenagers. It will discuss the importance of eating a balanced diet, the types of foods to include, and how to make healthier food choices. It will also provide tips for making healthy eating easier and more enjoyable for teenagers.

Eating healthy is especially important for growing teenagers. As teens continue to grow and undergo physical and emotional changes, it is important to ensure their diets provide them with all the essential nutrients their bodies need.

Chapter 1

Introduction to Healthy Eating for Teenagers

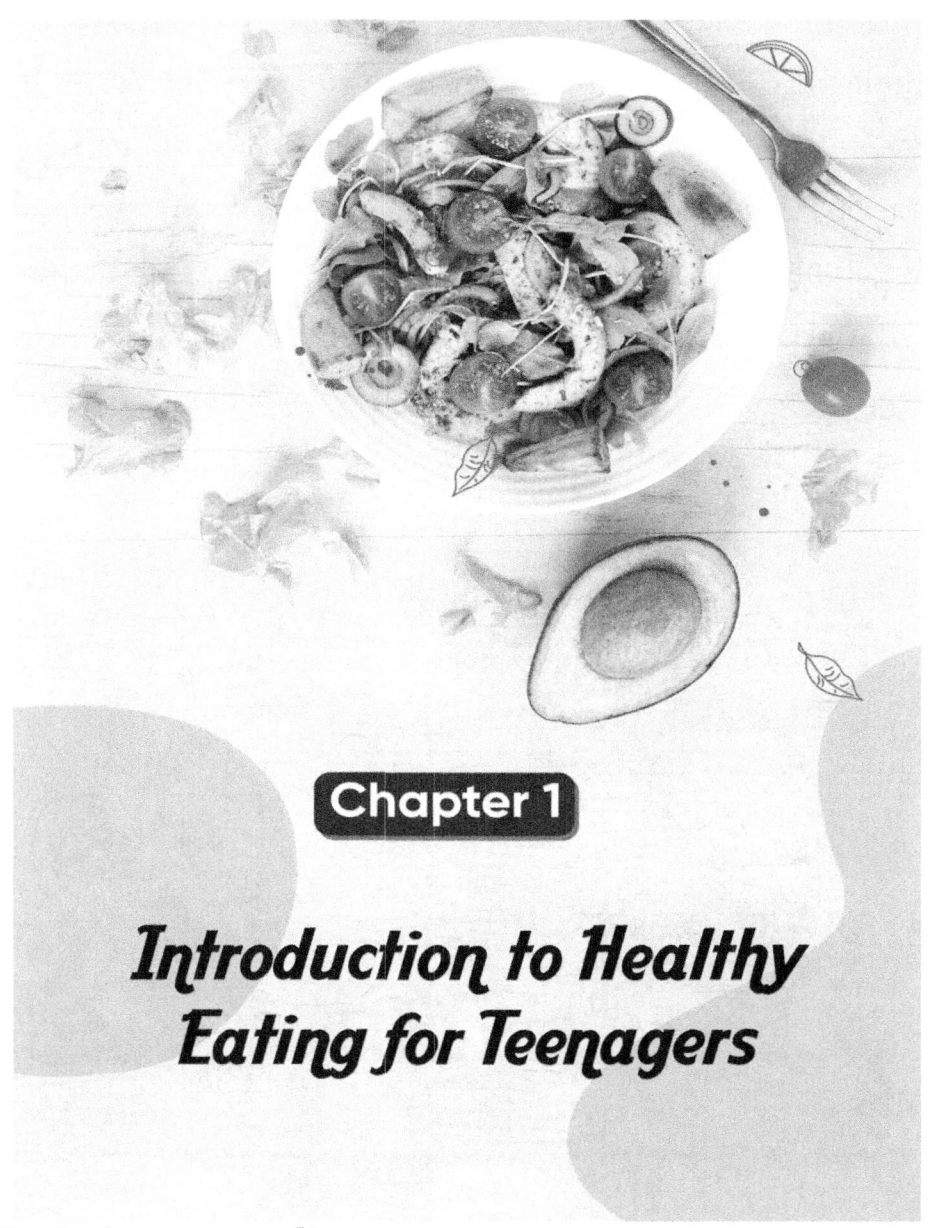

So, Let's get started!

Healthy eating during the teenage years is essential for proper growth and development. It is important to understand that the food choices teenagers make today can affect their health later in life. As teenagers grow, their need for certain nutrients and energy increases. To meet these needs, teenagers should focus on eating a variety of healthy foods, including lean proteins, vegetables, whole grains, and healthy fats. This chapter will provide an introduction to healthy eating for growing teenagers.

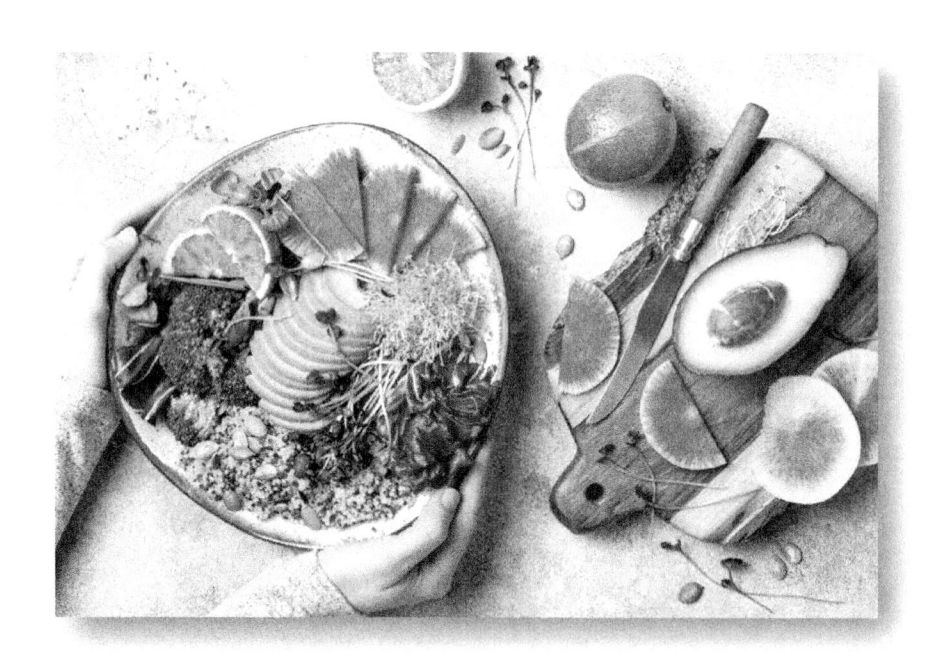

With the right guidance, teenagers can begin to develop a healthy lifestyle that will benefit them both now and in the future.

1.1 What is healthy food?

Healthy food gives them all the nutrients they need to stay healthy, feel well, and have plenty of energy.

Healthy food is not only good for their physical health but also for their mental and emotional health.

Healthy foods are fresh and natural, free from additives, preservatives, and artificial colors. It contains the right amount of carbohydrates, fats, proteins, vitamins, minerals, and antioxidants.

The best way to ensure they're eating healthily is to make them eat various kinds of food.

Have vegetables, salad, or fruit with every meal – it is packed with vitamins, minerals, and fiber that are good for a teen's health, help them feel full, and protect them from chronic diseases. Eat a variety of colors for the best mix of protective nutrients. At least five servings of vegetables, salad, and fruit are recommended for a healthy diet.

Cereals, rice, pasta, potatoes, and slices of bread are great energy sources. It's best to eat wholegrain versions as it contains fiber to keep their digestive system working well.

How much they need depends on their age, size, gender, and activity levels.

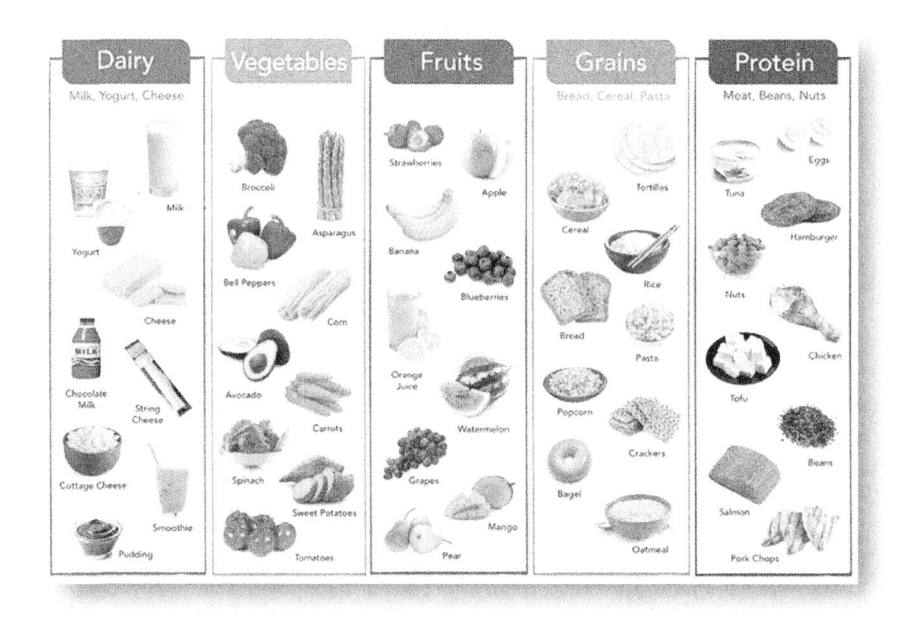

Milk, yogurt, and cheese provide calcium and protein. Calcium is needed for healthy bones throughout life. Choose reduced-fat or low-fat varieties, which provide the same amount of calcium and other nutrients with fewer calories and saturated fat.

Their body needs protein to support growth and maintain a healthy body, so it is needed every day. Meat, poultry, fish, eggs, beans, and nuts are good ways to include protein in their diet.

When preparing meat dishes, go for lean meats and poultry. Have fish at least twice a week – white fish on one day and oily fish on another. Oily fish provides essential omega-3 fats that keep their heart healthy.

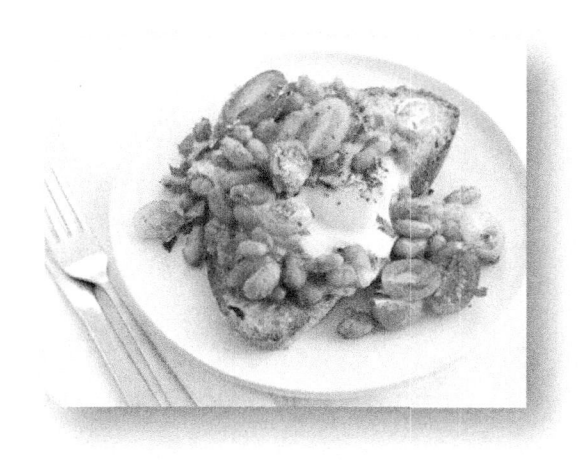

Beans and eggs are good choices for meat-free days.

Healthy fats are essential to a balanced diet but are only needed in very small amounts.

Low-fat spreads and vegetable oils such as rapeseed and olive oil are best. Saturated fats, found in hard fats like butter, can raise cholesterol levels.

Have healthy snacks like fruit, vegetables, low-fat dairy, and high-fiber cereals instead of snacks high in fat, sugar, and salts like sweets, cakes, and crisps.

It's easy to forget that drinks make up a big part of their diets. Water and milk are the healthiest

options, and sugary drinks are best avoided.

Variety is the key. Their body needs many different nutrients to stay healthy - no food or food group can provide all these. They don't have to get the balance right at every meal: try to balance out over the day or even the week.

Food planning can help them see what they're eating and make their choices healthier.

1.2 Why should teens eat healthy food?

Teenagers go through big physical changes in puberty. They need extra nutrition to fuel these physical changes, which means they need to eat healthy food.

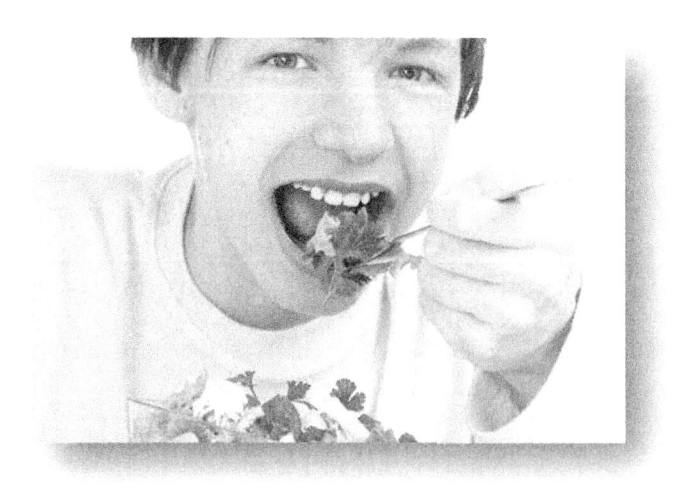

Their level of physical activity and stage of development determine exactly how much healthy food they need.

But you'll notice they have a bigger appetite, which is their body's way of telling them to eat more.

5 Reasons Why Teens Need to Eat Healthily?

When they are little kids, what goes onto their table and hence, into their mouths can be controlled. But once they are teens, they can make their own food. Despite this, one cannot insist on healthy meals in your home.

Home groceries should be planned by keeping delicious and nutritious snacks around that teens will want to eat.

Here's why helping them eat healthily is so important.

1. It keeps their complexion clearer.

Remember when you were a teen, and your biggest problem was a sudden zit?

It was the worst thing that could happen to you, aside from wondering if the person you liked returned your feelings.

With a zit, how could anyone like you? Times may have changed, but breakouts are still a bust for all teens. By eating healthy, a teen will have clearer and healthier skin.

2. It gives them better focus.

Empty calories from sugary treats or sodas provide zero nutrients. Yes, calories are needed for energy, but it's terrible for teens when they lack nutritional value.

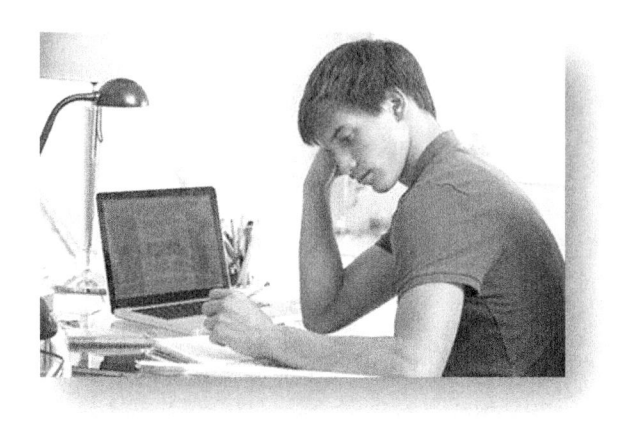

It leads to a lack of concentration, making their school work suffer. Fuel their minds and bodies properly with nutritious foods instead.

3. It gives them more energy for sports.

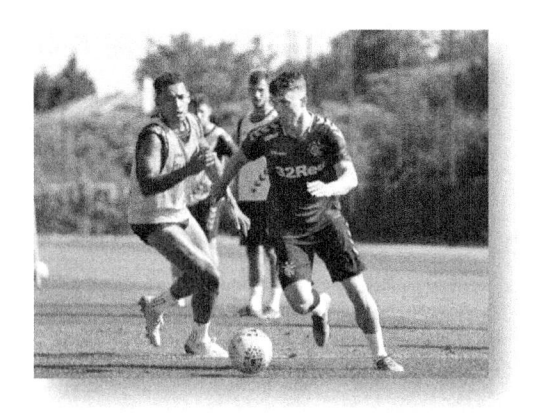

Whether a teen is on the football team, a cheerleader, or loves heading to the park with a skateboard, proper nutrition from healthy eating gives them the energy and strength to be physically active.

The more active they are, the healthier they will be overall.

4. It helps their immunity.

All kids love to fake sick to stay home from school. But when they're really sick, it's a different story. No one likes being sick in bed and feeling weak.

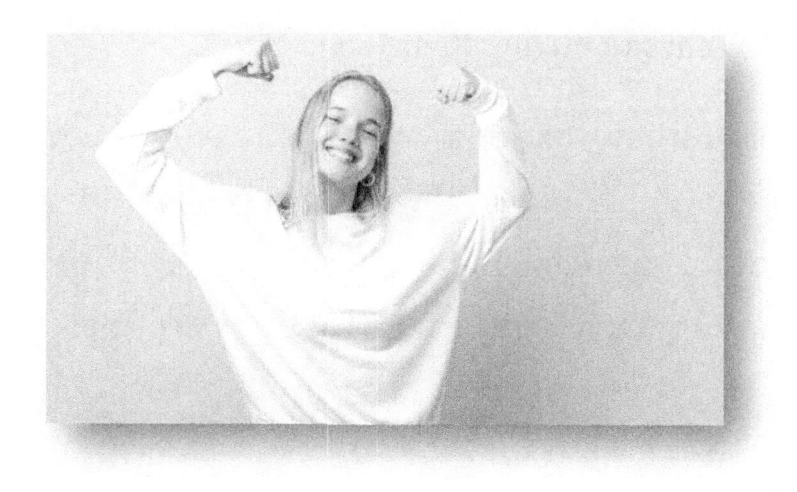

By nourishing them with good whole foods, you'll lessen the likelihood that they'll come down with something that will have them in bed for a week.

5. It helps them build good habits for adulthood.

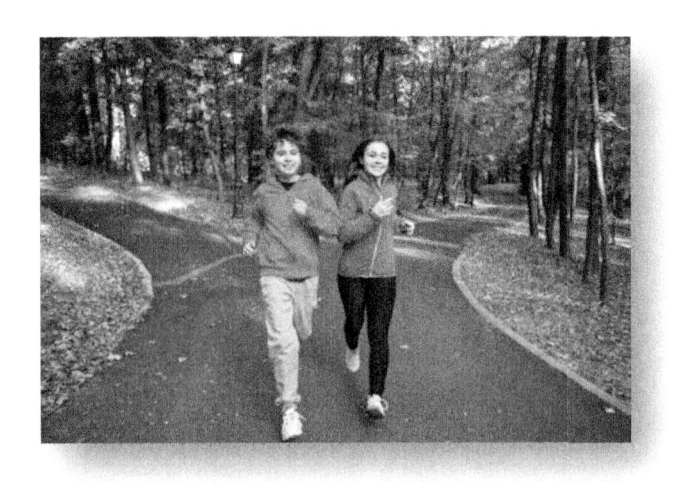

It won't be long before your teen is considered an official adult. Set a good pattern of habits by encouraging healthy eating at home. Once they're living on their own, they'll be more likely to make smart choices when it comes to buying their food.

Kids learn from what they see us do. Even teens who act as if they'd rather see off their own arms instead of being seen with us in public! Make healthy eating a priority at home to keep teenagers healthy for years to come!

1.3 How to introduce healthy eating habits for teenagers?

With the rising rates of obesity, the need to instill healthy eating habits in teenagers has become increasingly important.

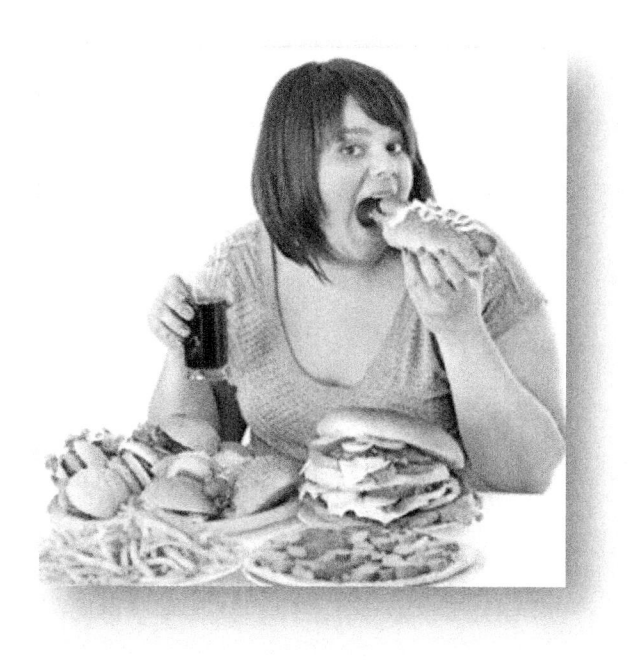

Teenagers are at a critical age where they are transitioning into adulthood and are more likely to be influenced by their peers and the media.

To help teenagers develop healthy eating habits, it is important to provide them with education, support, and positive reinforcement.

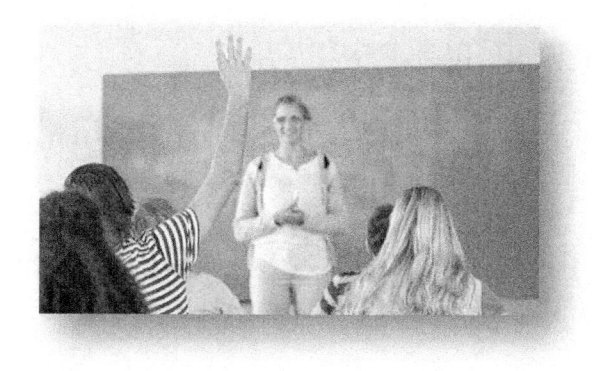

Educate: Provide teenagers with information about healthy eating and nutrition.

Educate them on the benefits of eating a balanced diet with plenty of fruits, vegetables, whole grains, and lean proteins.

Teach them about portion sizes and the importance of limiting processed and sugary foods.

Support: Make healthy eating easy and accessible for teenagers.

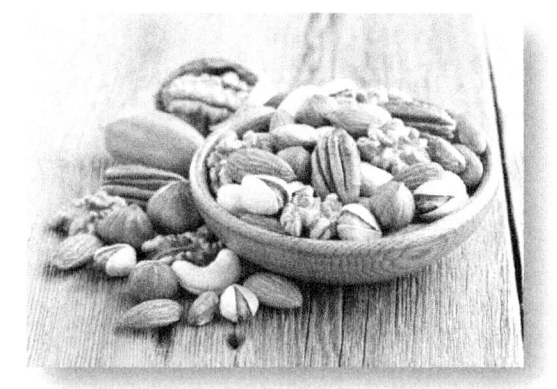

Keep healthy snacks in the house, such as nuts, fruits, and vegetables, and encourage them to make healthy choices.

Create a shopping list for them with healthy options and encourage them to help with meal planning.

Reinforce: Reinforce positive behaviors and provide positive feedback when teenagers make healthy choices. Avoid punishing them for unhealthy choices, and provide them with incentives and rewards for making healthy choices.

By following these strategies, parents can help introduce healthy eating habits in teenagers and set them up for a lifetime of healthy eating.

Chapter 2

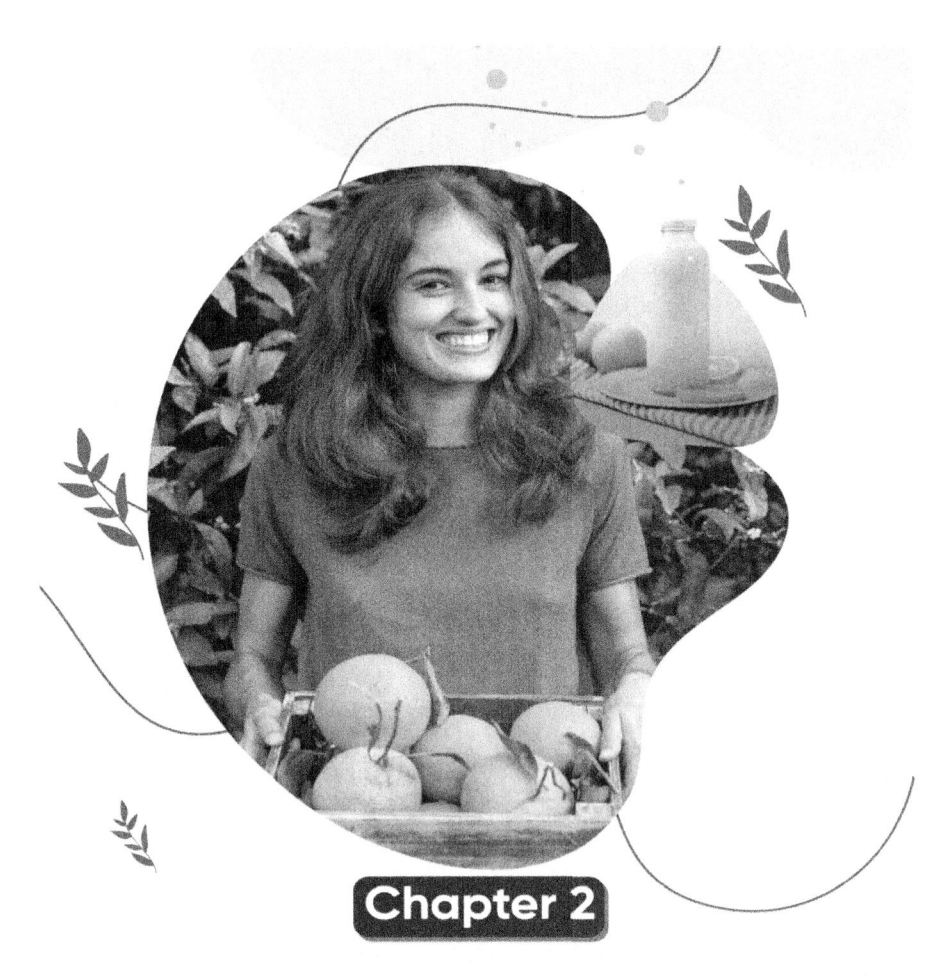

Identifying Nutritional Needs for Teenagers

Adolescence is a time of tremendous growth, both physically and mentally. As teens navigate their way through this critical time in their lives, they need to understand how to meet their nutritional needs. A balanced diet is essential to their physical and mental health and their educational success.

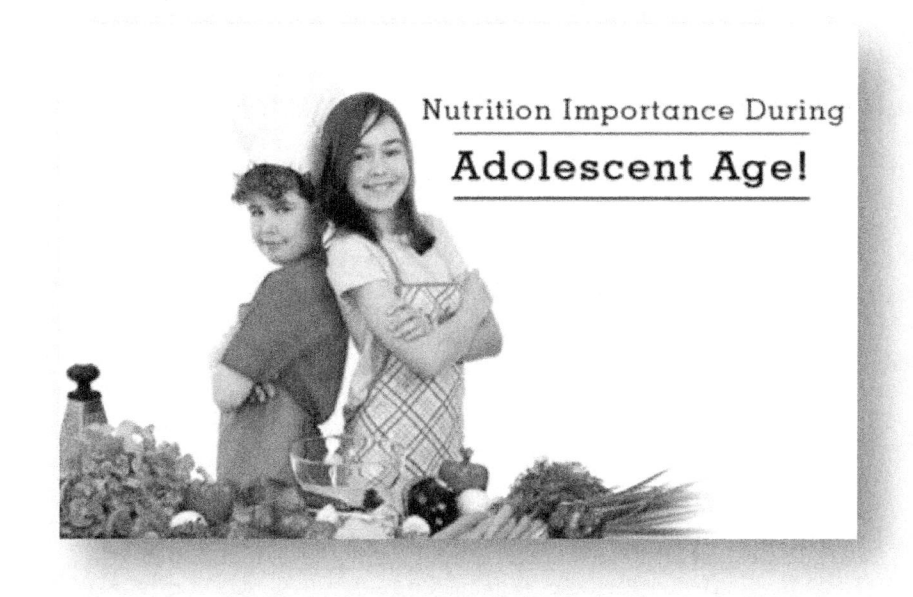

In this chapter, we will explore the dietary needs of teenagers, the foods they should be eating to meet those needs, and the importance of creating healthy eating habits.

We will also discuss ways to identify and address teens' nutritional deficiencies.

By understanding the nutritional needs of teenagers and providing them with the necessary tools to make healthy decisions, we can ensure that they have the best chance of success.

2.1 Instigate what the nutritional needs are in teenagers.

Healthy habits like eating breakfast every day and not skipping meals should be emphasized. Parents who want their children to make their own eating choices should provide plenty of support and healthy meals at home. Adolescents need more calories, calcium, zinc, protein, iron, and most vitamins.

Calories

Adolescents' energy needs depend on BMR, activity level, and the need to stimulate pubertal development.

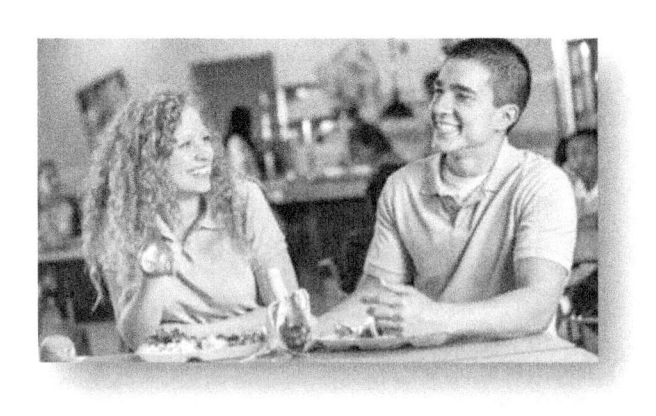

For teenagers, this means consuming more calories to keep up with their increased activity and development.

Teenage guys need more calories since they are larger and heavier than their female counterparts.

To achieve these nutritional needs, teenagers should eat lean protein sources, low-fat dairy products, whole grains, vegetables, and fruits.

A surge in appetite around the age of ten in girls and twelve in boys foreshadows the growth spurt of puberty. How much of a surge? Mom and Dad might want to oil the hinges on the refrigerator door and start stockpiling a small cache of their favorite snacks underneath the bed.

Calories are the measurement used to express the energy delivered by food. The body demands more calories during early adolescence than at any other time of life.

Boys require an average of 2,800 calories per day.

Girls require an average of 2,200 calories per day.

Typically, the ravenous hunger starts to wane once a child has stopped growing, though not always. Kids who are big and tall or participate in physical activity will still need increased energy into late adolescence.

During middle and late adolescence, girls eat roughly 25% fewer calories per day than boys do; consequently, they are more likely to be deficient in vitamins and minerals.

Protein

During the teenage development surge, protein is essential for maintaining muscular mass.

Females 11 to 14 years old have a greater protein demand per unit of height than males 15 to 18 years old.

The average teenager daily needs between 45 and 60 grams of protein. Teenagers often consume chicken, steak, eggs, and dairy products to achieve this protein requirement. Other good protein sources include nuts, soy foods, beans, and tofu.

Of the three nutrients, we're least concerned about protein. Not because it isn't important—50% of our body weight is made up of protein—but because adolescents in the United States get twice as much protein as they need.

The densest sources of protein include teenage favorites such as:

- Beef
- Chicken

- Turkey
- Pork
- Fish
- Eggs
- Cheese

Carbohydrates

Carbohydrates, found in starches and sugars, get converted into the body's main fuel: the simple sugar glucose.

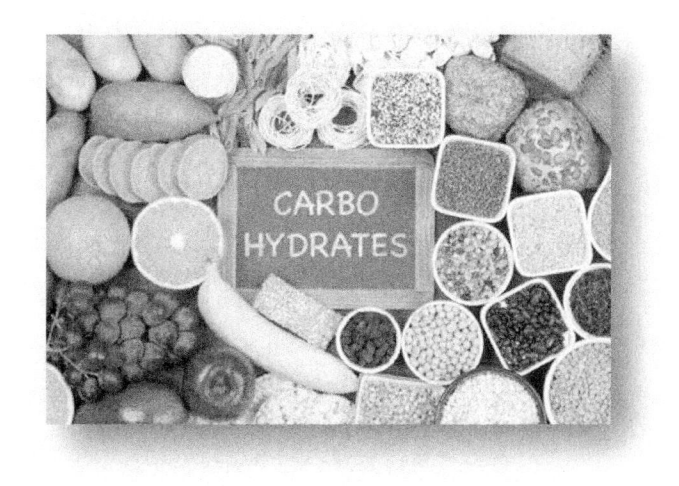

Not all carbs are created equal, however. In planning meals, we want to push complex-carbohydrate foods and go easy on simple carbohydrates.

Complex carbs provide sustained energy; that's why you often see marathon runners and other athletes downing big bowls of pasta before competing.

As a bonus, many starches deliver fiber and assorted nutrients too. They are truly foods of substance: filling yet low in fat.

Most nutritionists recommend that complex carbohydrates make up 50% to 60% of a teenager's caloric intake.

Simple carbs, on the other hand, seduce us with their sweet taste and a brief burst of energy but have little else to offer and should be minimized in the diet.

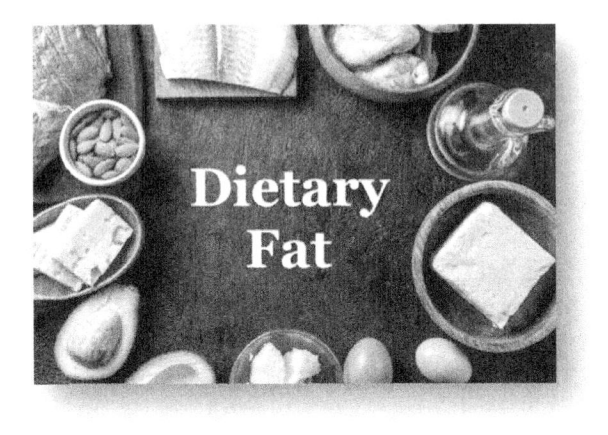

Dietary Fat

Fat should make up no more than 30% of the diet. Fat supplies energy and assists the body in absorbing the fat-soluble vitamins: A, D, E, and K. But these benefits must be considered next to its many adverse effects on health.

A teenager who indulges in a fat-heavy diet will put on weight, even if active. It would take a workout befitting an Olympic athlete to burn off excess fat calories day after day.

Fatty foods contain cholesterol, a waxy substance that can clog an artery and eventually cause it to harden. The danger of atherosclerosis is that the blockage will affect one of the blood vessels leading to the heart or the brain, setting off a heart attack or a stroke.

Although these life-threatening events usually don't strike until later in adulthood, the time to start practicing prevention is now by reducing the amount of fat in your family's diet.

Dietary fat contains varying proportions of three types:

Monounsaturated fat —the healthiest kind; found in olives and olive oil; peanuts, peanut oil, and peanut butter; cashews; walnuts and walnut oil; and canola oil.

Polyunsaturated fat—found in corn oil, safflower oil, sunflower oil, soybean oil, cottonseed oil, and sesame-seed oil.

Saturated fat —is the most cholesterol-laden of the three; found in meat and dairy products like beef, pork, lamb, butter, cheese, cream, egg yolks, coconut oil, and palm oil.

You want to limit your teen's saturated fat intake to no more than 10% of their total daily calories. The other 20% of daily calories from dietary fat should come equally from the two unsaturated kinds of fat, which are contained mainly in plant oils.

If your teens eat many packaged and processed foods, remember to read the food labels. You may be surprised to see how much fat, sugar, and salt (sodium) are in their daily foods. And almost all packaged goods that contain fat are likely to have partially hydrogenated fat because it has a longer shelf life.

Vitamins and Minerals

A well-rounded diet based on the USDA guidelines should deliver sufficient amounts of all the essential vitamins and minerals.

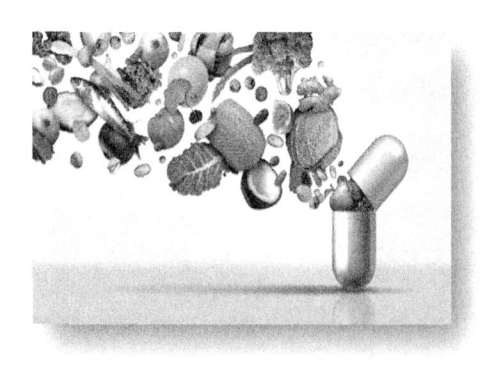

Adolescents often need to catch up to their daily calcium, iron, zinc, and vitamin D quotas.

Unless blood tests and a pediatrician's evaluation reveal a specific deficiency, it's preferable to obtain nutrients from food instead of from dietary supplements.

Vitamin A, B6, E, D, C, and folic acid deficiencies are common among teenagers. On the other hand, adolescents who consume the recommended daily allowance of nutrients do not suffer from vitamin deficiencies.

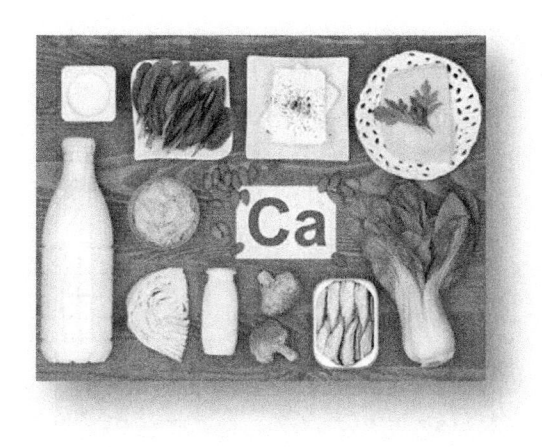

Calcium

During adolescence, bone mass reaches a maximum of 45 percent. For this reason, children must have enough calcium in their diets. One thousand one hundred thirty-five milligrams of calcium daily is recommended for adolescents between 9 and 18.

According to the American Academy of Pediatrics, milk, cheese, yogurt, calcium-fortified drinks, and cereals are the best sources of calcium for teenagers.

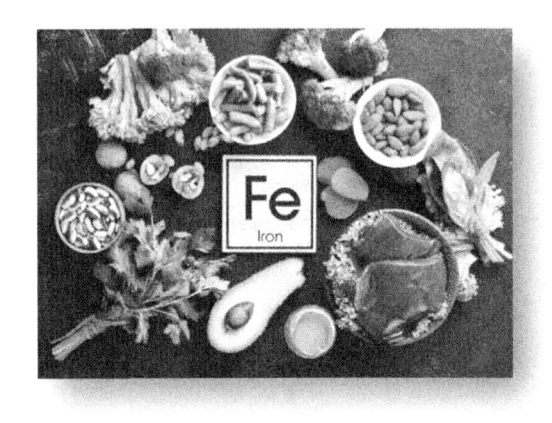

Iron

A lack of iron in circulation may lead to anemia, which can be fatal.

Male adolescents need 12 mg of iron daily, whereas female adolescents need 15 mg.

Eating a wide variety of iron-rich foods is a good idea to ensure you're getting enough.

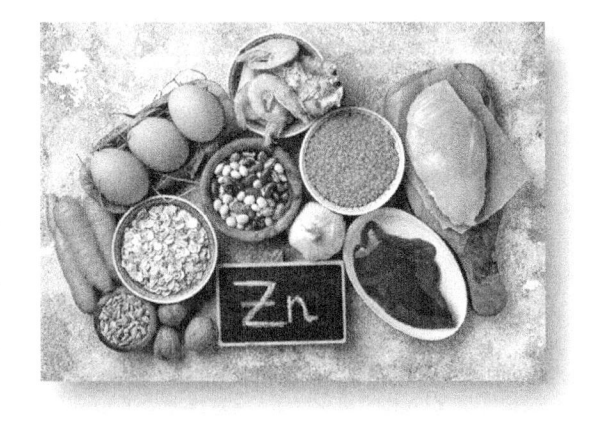

Zinc

Gene expression and protein synthesis are dependent on zinc. It's critical in adolescence since it aids in physical and sexual development.

There is a link between zinc deficiency in males and stunted growth.

Fish, shellfish, and red meat are excellent sources of zinc, as are complete grains and legumes. Breakfast cereals enriched with zinc are also a good source of zinc. Its insufficiency is a common problem among adolescent vegetarians, particularly those who avoid animal products.

Teens develop physically and socially throughout adolescence. As a result, proper nutrition throughout this time should not be underestimated. Adolescent eating decisions will have an impact on both their current and future health throughout this time.

2.2 Find out why nutrition is required for teenagers.

The teenage years are one of the most exciting moments in life. During the teenage, a body undergoes hormonal changes, weight gain or loss, growth, and physical changes. Rapid growth and development need increased nutrition and energy intake.

Therefore, it is crucial to learn the importance of nutrition during the teenage years.

Why is it important to understand the nutritional problems of an adolescent?

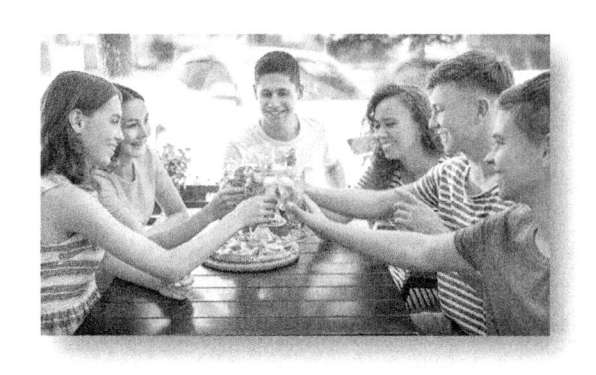

During adolescence, a person's nutritional and dietary demands alter due to changes in the body.

Teenagers are growing more self-reliant and making a maximum number of eating choices for themselves. Growth spurts and increased appetites are common among teenagers.

They need nutritious diets to keep up with their flourishing bodies. When compared to younger children, teenagers consume more meals out than at home.

Peer pressure also has a major impact on them. Since they find it convenient, adolescents consume too much junk food, such as sodas, fast food, and processed meals.

In addition, dieting is a major worry for many teenagers. Peer pressure might lead girls to try to lose weight by cutting down on what they consume. Both boys and females may do dieting to "make weight" for an athletic or social event.

How does nutrition affect adolescent development?

Adolescents require nutritional counseling to maintain healthy lifestyles, minimize weight-related issues, reduce illness risk, and ensure proper development and growth.

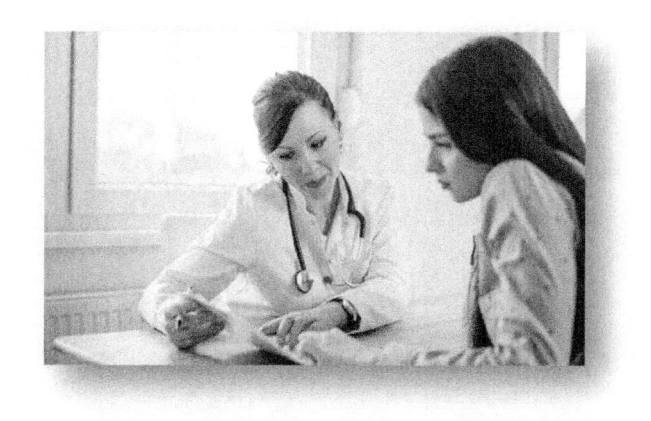

Eating healthily in moderation and engaging in regular exercise may help avoid weight gain, iron deficiency, anemia, and poor bone mineralization.

Obesity or being overweight throughout youth raises the chance of developing type 2 diabetes later in life. As a result, eating habits developed throughout adolescence may have a long-term impact on the likelihood of developing chronic conditions, including heart disease, osteoporosis, and cancer in later life.

As adolescence progresses, so does the need for energy and other nutrients.

2.3 What is the role of parents in ensuring adequate nutrition?

Parental nutrition knowledge and attitudes are fundamental to their children's food knowledge. The role of parental behavior in the development of food preferences is considered.

Food preferences develop from genetically determined predispositions to like sweet and salty flavors and to dislike bitter and sour tastes.

Food aversions can be learned in one trial if discomfort follows consumption. There is a predisposition to learn to like foods with high-energy density.

However, from birth, genetic predispositions are modified by experience, and in this context, parents play a particularly important role during the early years.

Parental style is a critical factor in the development of food preferences. Children are more likely to eat in emotionally positive atmospheres.

Siblings, peers, and parents can be role models to encourage novel-tasting foods. Repeated exposure to initially disliked foods can break down resistance.

The offering of low-energy-dense foods allows the child to balance energy intake.

Restricting access to particular foods increases rather than decreases preference. Forcing a teen to eat food will decrease their liking for that food.

Traditionally, educational strategies have typically involved attempts to impart basic nutritional information.

Given the limited ability of information to induce changes in behavior, an alternative strategy would be to teach parents about teen's development in the hope that understanding the characteristic innate tendencies and developmental stages can be used to teach healthy food preferences.

Parental style

Parents often have a policy of manipulating the availability of certain foods, either for a perceived health gain or as a reward or punishment. The question is whether such approaches achieve their intended consequences.

Food as a reward

Offering one food as a reward for eating another is a common strategy; teens need to eat up their vegetables to have a dessert. The pattern is clear.

The preference for the food used as the reward increases, and there is a decrease in the preference for distasteful food. When teens are rewarded for eating disliked food, this leads to a decline in their preference.

Rather than increasing the probability that a desirable food was consumed, the approach had the opposite effect. It became more unlikely that the child ate the food.

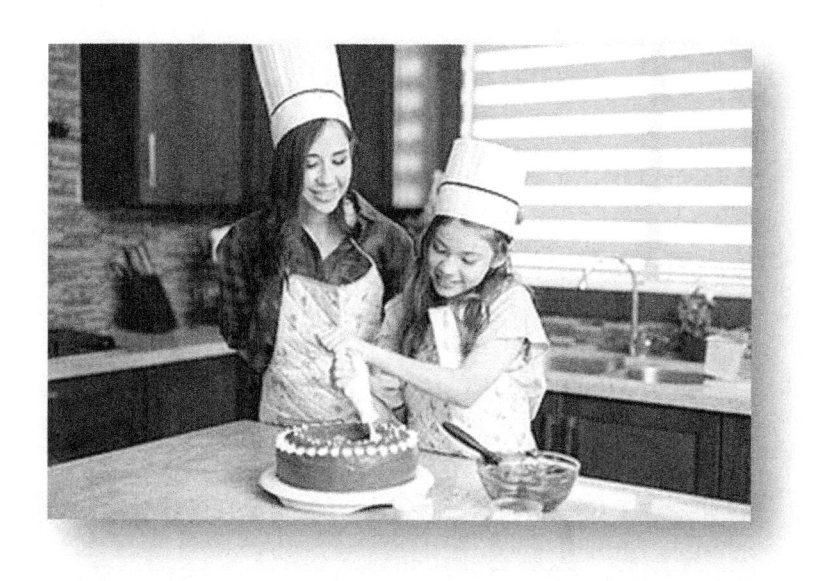

In a negative context, using food initially disliked to gain access to something pleasurable is not helpful. Foods are sometimes paired with parental attention and rewards.

When teens are offered food items that were initially neither liked nor disliked but were used as rewards over six weeks or associated with parental attention, the liking for these foods increases. It is easy to generalize this finding to real-life situations.

High-fat and sweet items such as chocolate are used repeatedly in positive contexts.

For example, they are given to those we like, on special occasions, or to say thank you. The consumption of already pleasurable items is, in this way, reinforced. If teenagers are given foods as rewards for approved behavior, their preference for those foods is enhanced.

Cultural influences

The best predictor of food preferences is knowledge of your cultural group. 'Grazing' rather than eating meals and the desire for convenience foods are increasingly common and associated with decreased cooking skills. Fewer meals are eaten in the home, and fewer meals are eaten as a family group, decreasing the opportunity for the parents to offer a model of healthy eating.

In America, 46% of expenditure is spent on food consumed outside the home, with 34% of the food expenditure on fast foods. American adolescents consumed 27–30% of their meals away from home, with 18% as a comparable figure for preschoolers.

Fast-food restaurants accounted for more than half of these meals.

In American adolescents, the frequency of using fast-food restaurants was positively associated with total energy intake and the percent of energy coming from fat: it was also negatively associated with the consumption of fruit and vegetables. The related problem is that meals eaten outside the home tend to have a higher energy density and are served in large portions.

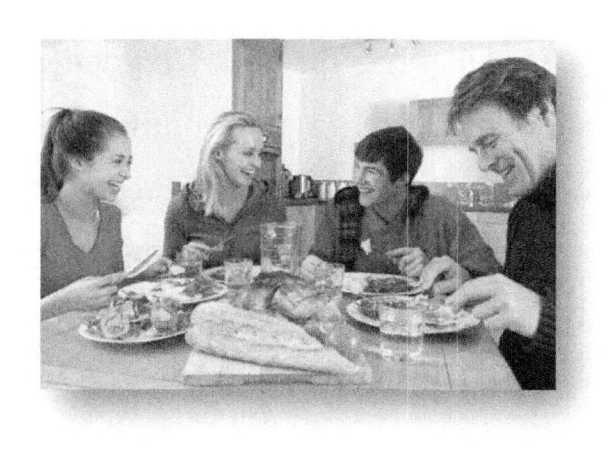

Eating dinner with the family is a less frequent phenomenon, particularly among adolescents. Those eating more often as a family consumed more fruit and vegetables and less fat.

Systematic differences in the diets of American teens are related to the frequency with that they watch television while eating. Frequent watching television during a meal was associated with 5% more of their energy intake coming from pizza, salty snacks, and soda and 5% less from fruit, vegetables, and juices.

Watching television was associated with lower consumption of carbohydrates and greater caffeine consumption.

Many factors may lead to this association. Those were watching television will be exposed to more advertising, which may also encourage eating quick-prepared snack foods rather than more elaborate meals.

Parents whose children watch more television tended to choose easy-to-prepare foods because the children ate them without complaining. There was evidence that watching television was associated with eating some foods that were not normally advertised, suggesting that this activity is a marker for parental attitudes toward providing their children's meals.

Over recent decades, there have been marked cultural changes in the nature and patterning of meals, where and with whom they are eaten. Each change brings with it implications for the diet.

Nutritional education for parents

Family involvement is an important element in effective nutrition education for school-going teenagers.

Schools should use any of the following strategies to involve parents in the nutrition education of their children:

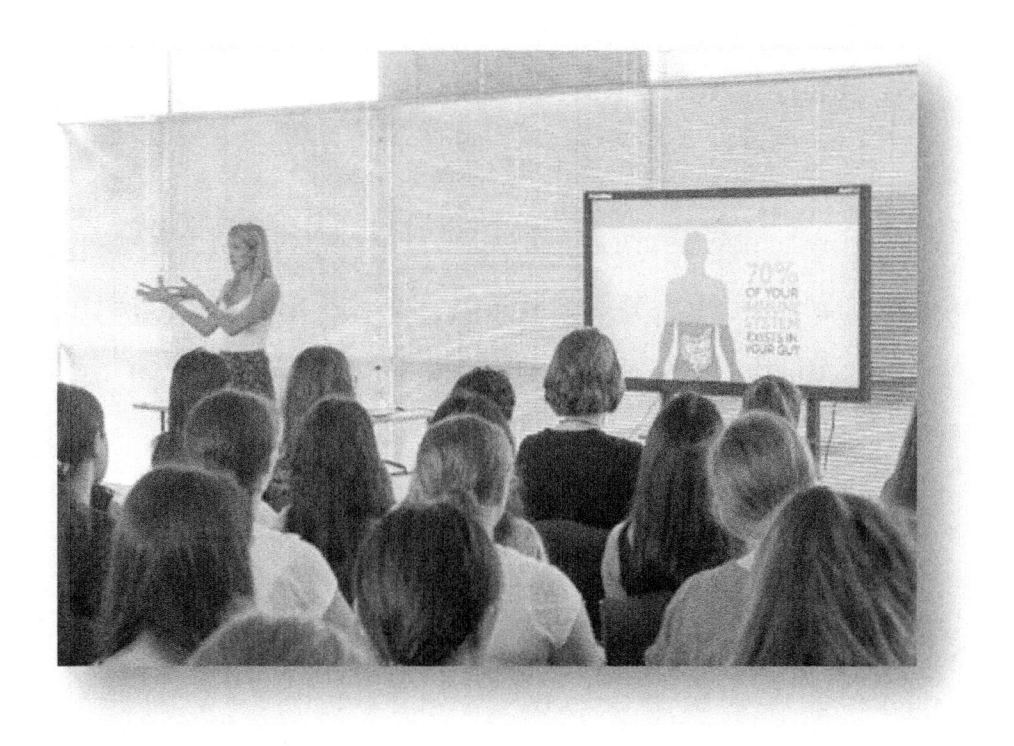

- Including parents in homework assignments.
- Sending home educational materials to help parents learn about nutrition or teach their children about nutrition.
- Inviting parents to attend nutrition classes.
- Inviting parents to attend special events, such as School Lunch Week or tasting parties.

- Inviting parents in nutrition-related careers to speak to the class.
- Asking parents to give in-class demonstrations.
- Asking parents to send healthful snacks to school.
- Offering nutrition workshops or screening services for parents.

With the exception of asking parents to send healthful snacks, a majority of teachers reported that they or their schools used these strategies to a small extent to make teens eat healthily.

Chapter 3

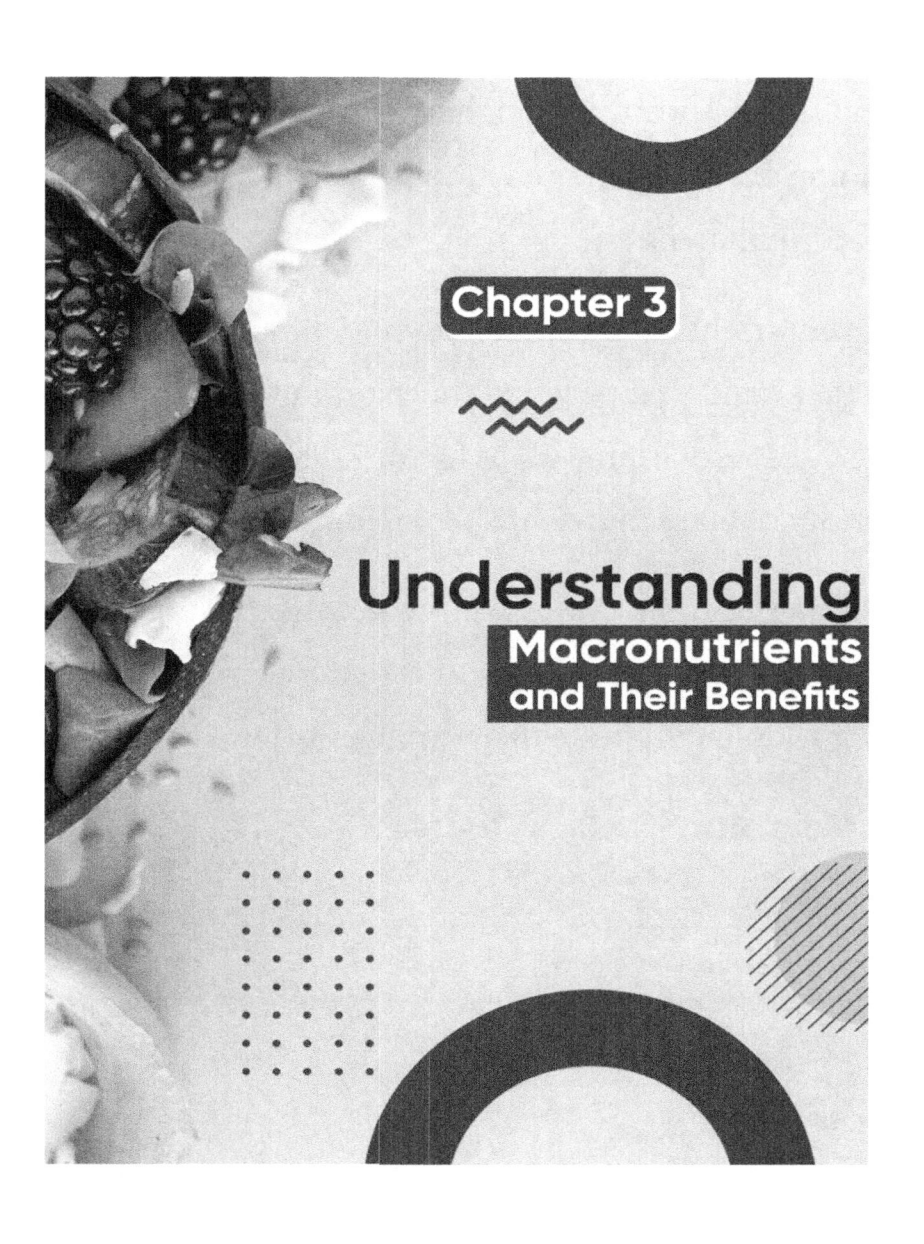

Understanding Macronutrients and Their Benefits

Macronutrients, or macros, provide energy for the body and help prevent disease. They are required in large amounts for the body to function properly and to maintain a healthy weight. Macronutrients are the building blocks of our diets and are needed for growth and development.

Macronutrients are available in many food sources, but it can take time to determine the right amount to consume. There are also a number of factors that can influence the quantity of macronutrients people may need.

In this chapter, we will see the importance of macronutrients in the body, different macronutrient diets, and how to incorporate macronutrients for a healthy diet.

3.1 Macronutrients: What Are They?

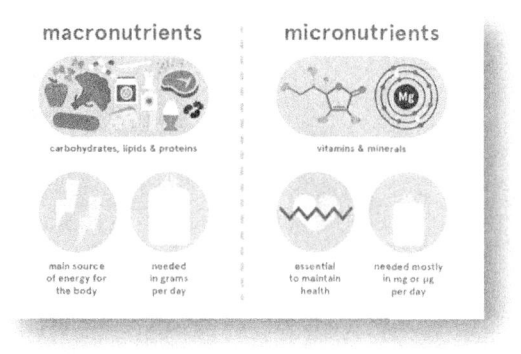

There are two main categories to consider: macronutrients and micronutrients. Micronutrients are mostly vitamins and minerals and are equally important but consumed very small amounts.

We generally get our micronutrients along with macronutrients. Some may also include other nutrients that people require in large amounts, such as water.

Most of the body's energy and calories come from macronutrients. Each type of macronutrient has its benefits and purpose in maintaining a healthy body. The exact amount of each macronutrient a person requires may vary based on individual factors such as weight, age, and preexisting health conditions.

Importance of macronutrients

Each type of macronutrient performs an important role in keeping the body healthy. For optimum health, people typically require a balance of macronutrients.

Carbohydrates:

Carbohydrates are a preferred energy source for several body tissues and the primary energy source for the brain. The body can break carbohydrates into glucose, which moves from the bloodstream into the body's cells and allows them to function.

Carbohydrates are important for muscle contraction during intense exercise. Even at rest, carbohydrates enable the body to perform vital functions such as maintaining body temperature, keeping the heart beating, and digesting food.

Protein:

Protein consists of long chains of compounds called amino acids. These are essential in developing, repairing, and maintaining body tissues. Protein is present in every body cell, and adequate protein intake keeps the muscles, bones, and tissues healthy. Protein also plays a vital role in many bodily processes, such as aiding the immune system, biochemical reactions, and providing structure and support for cells.

Fats:

Fats are an important part of the diet that can also provide the body with energy. While some types of dietary fats may be healthier than others, they are an essential part of the diet and play a role trusted Source in hormone production, cell growth, energy storage, and the absorption of important vitamins.

How much to consume?

The following percentages of macronutrients are good for health and provide essential nutrition:

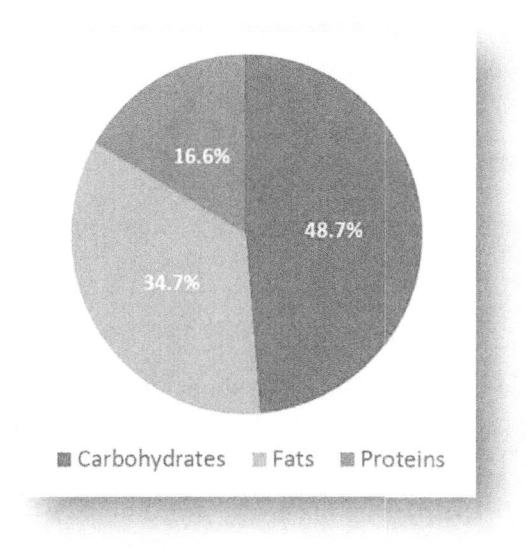

45–65% carbohydrates

20–35% fats

10–35% protein

People's calorie and macro requirements can vary due to age, sex, and in women whether they are pregnant. Additionally, other factors that can influence a person's macro requirements can include:

- current weight
- fitness goals
- existing health conditions
- current muscle mass

And about the food sources, we have already discussed them in the above chapters. (Chapter 2)

3.2 What are the benefits of macronutrients?

All micronutrients are extremely important to teenagers for the proper functioning of their bodies.

Consuming an adequate amount of the different vitamins and minerals is key to optimal health and may even help fight disease.

This is because micronutrients are part of nearly every process in your body. Moreover, certain vitamins and minerals can act as antioxidants.

Antioxidants may protect against cell damage associated with certain diseases, including cancer, Alzheimer's, and heart disease.

For example, an adequate dietary intake of vitamins A and C helps lower the risk of some types of cancer.

Getting enough of some vitamins may also help prevent Alzheimer's disease.

Adequate dietary intake of vitamins E, C, and A is associated with a 24%, 17%, and 12% reduced risk of developing Alzheimer's, respectively.

Certain minerals may also play a role in preventing and fighting disease.

Low blood levels of selenium to a higher risk of heart disease. The risk of heart disease decreased by 24% when blood concentrations of selenium increased by 50%.

Additionally, adequate calcium intake decreases the risk of death from heart disease and all other causes.

Consuming enough of all micronutrients — especially those with antioxidant properties — provides ample health benefits.

However, it's unclear whether consuming more than the recommended amounts of certain micronutrients from foods or supplements offers additional benefits.

3.3 Combinations and timings of macronutrients.

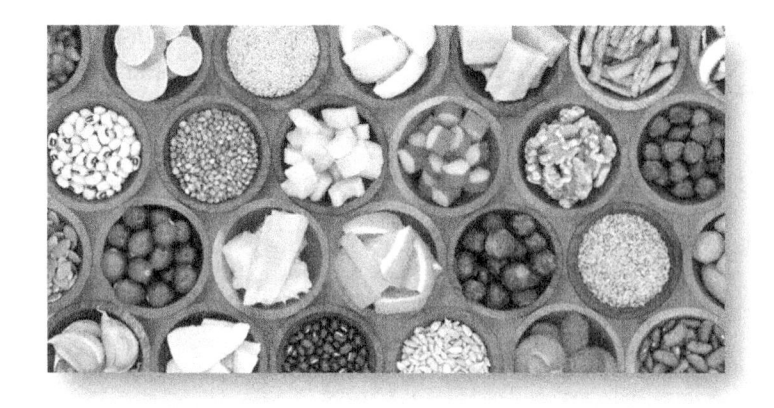

The timeless debate of optimal macronutrient combinations.

While not the end all, be all of the debates or appearance-altering factors, the combination in which you eat your macronutrients can negatively impact your physique. It only creates confusion and disillusion around what foods to eat, when to eat them, and in which company of other foods.

We don't need any more unnecessary disillusion and confusion. We need results. And we'll be damned if we are not the coach to deliver you said these results.

Over the course of this chapter, we're going to dig into and understand the application and effects of different macronutrient combinations.

Use this information at your own risk: the resultant gains may be larger than ever imagined.

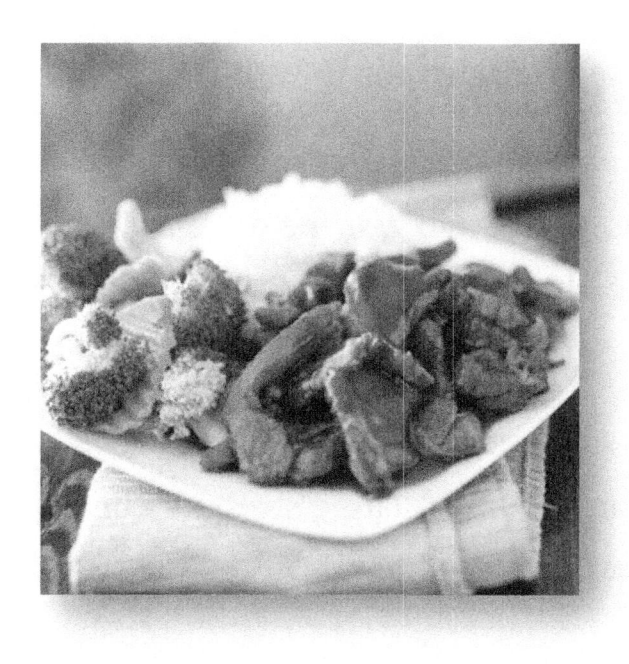

Protein and Carbs

Optimal Timing: Post-workout

Taking in a meal based on protein and carbs with only trace fats helps kickstart muscle protein synthesis.

Why: Protein and carbohydrate-based meals are some of the best and tastiest meals out there. How can you turn down a massive rice bowl of perfectly stir-fried mushrooms, onions, and peppers topped with juicy steak slices?

After training, especially with the goal of building muscle, replenishing your intra-muscular glycogen becomes quite important. This replenishment can be readily accomplished by taking in foods such as rice, potatoes, pasta, or your favorite flavor of frozen yogurt and waffles.

Why Not: Naturally, as with any nutritional method, dietary freedom doesn't work well for everyone.

The resulting insulin spike can make some people very sleepy and lethargic. This could also be a sign that you have had too many carbs and may want to dial back your serving size next time around.

One can reduce daily carbohydrate intake, look at lifestyle, and place focus on modulating stress in a healthy spot for their body internally and physically.

It's much more important that your body handles nutrients appropriately than it is for you to get your daily dose of sweets.

Protein and Fat

Optimal Timing: Breaking the fast and meals earlier in your day. Think of meals such as bacon and eggs, a turkey patty, and nut butter or chicken lettuce breakfast 'tacos.'

Why: Protein- and fat-based meals may promote greater fatty acid metabolism and resultant fat burning as there is hype in every generation that they wait to introduce carbs into a day.

By allowing fasting blood glucose to stay low, minimizing spikes in insulin, and not taking in carbs, you keep your physique in a healthy and happy state of fat burning.

Besides, bacon, egg, and avocado are a pretty damn tasty combination to kick off your day.

Why Not: Carbs are delicious, enjoyable, and productive for muscle growth. Not being one to enjoy being forever hungry, teens must prefer to get a vast amount of calories from carbs.

Too many of these meals can easily push them into an unwanted surplus or erase their deficit due to fats being over twice as calorically dense as carbs. This means you are not allowing "open season" on fats, regardless of how "healthy" they may be.

Protein, Fat, and Carbs

Optimal timing: Pre-workout, refeeds/cheat meals

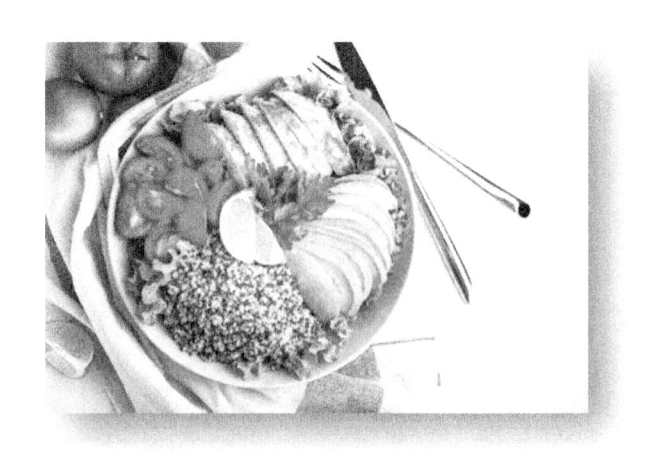

Why: It's important to have a healthy supply of amino acids circulating in your blood. The more you minimize any chance of tapping into muscle tissue for fuel, the better. Doing so is important for maintaining muscle protein synthesis and preventing catabolizing precious muscle tissue.

Teenagers should have the knowledge of good or bad. So it must be a big no from their side to Cold sweats, energy tanks, and poor contractions; everything becomes twice as heavy.

Why Not: As with anything truly delicious, these meals can be a double-edged sword. Unless wisely made at home, many of these meals are very calorically dense due to LOTS of fat. That said, this does make them near-perfect for free meals.

If a teen is lean or depleted enough, they'll notice improved vascularity, energy, and muscle fullness after eating such a meal. But if you're to have that every day? You'll be digging yourself into a hole when it comes to fat loss.

Again, these meals are best approached with precision and made at home unless you've got a planned refeed on deck.

Carbs Before Bed — Massing Phase

First of all, eating carbs after 6 pm will NOT make you fat (unless it puts you into a surplus).

There isn't some magical insulin fairy who sits by the pool all day waiting for 6 pm to hit. Then when 6 pm comes, said fairy gets up and decides that everything you eat between now and 8 am will be stored as fat. This is a simple-minded fabrication.

Why: The dopamine rush from ingesting carbs allows the body and mind to relax. This is perfect for before bed, as it promotes your pineal gland to secrete melatonin. Aside from supporting a healthy circadian rhythm, melatonin relates it will help you fall asleep and improve your overall sleep quality.

If you train bright and early, eating a bushel of carbohydrates the night before will load your muscles with glycogen that can be used as fuel to push you.

If you take in a moderately sized bolus of carbohydrates 60-90 minutes before bed, you should hit the sheets in a perfect balance between being hungry and overstuffed.

Why Not: As with nearly every nuance of nutrition, each technique and combination method have two sides. Eating a bolus of carbs before bed may make you sleep, ultimately affecting a teen's studies.

However, if you overdo it (easy to do at night), eat something that irritates your gut, or don't have sufficient digestive firepower, that carries a feast before bed could result in you waking up bloated and full. Waking up full and bloated before is a challenging experience.

The Final Reps and Your Takeaways

Ultimately, you must mess around for a while and figure out what works for your teen and when it works best. As well as consider the context of your goals when deciding how and when to lay out your macros.

That may be different from what you wanted to hear, but as with any sound nutrition advice, things become very individual and must be treated as such.

Here's what you need to take away:

Different macronutrient combinations can each have their own physiological effects, advantages, and disadvantages. Learn how to use each combination to suit a teenager's body needs.

Of all the macronutrients, carbohydrates have the power to do the most damage and the best for everyone's body.

Dopamine can have a powerful impact on one's physique and recovery. Manipulate nutrition for teens wisely and take total advantage of it.

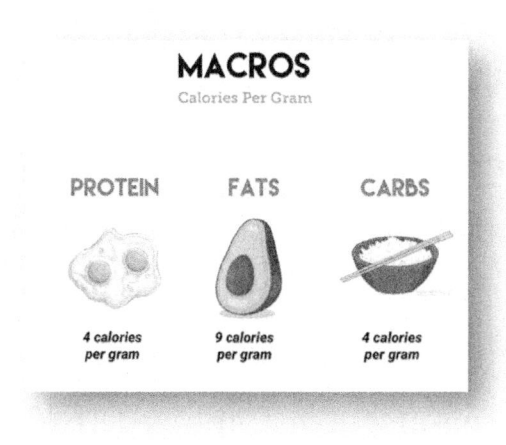

3.4 Why is it essential to have macronutrients for teenagers?

Nutrition during the teenage years is of paramount importance because good nutrition aids growth, development, and learning. While teenagers should avoid restrictive diets or those that limit certain food groups or macronutrients, eating a healthy diet with a good balance of protein, carbohydrates, and fats is key. Help teenagers to improve their diets by encouraging them to make healthy choices.

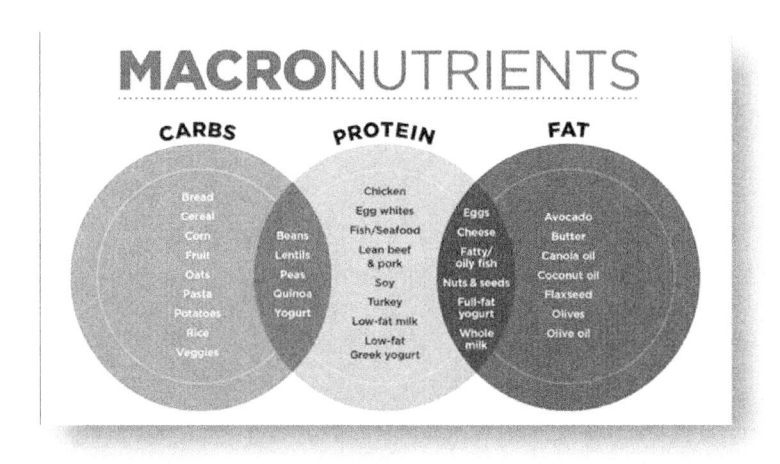

Recently, the dietary macronutrient proportion in the diet and food selection patterns of children and adolescents affected body composition and metabolic status.

A short-term (12-week) randomized clinical trial for weight loss performed in obese adolescents showed that both a low-fat diet (55% carbohydrate; 20% protein; 25% fat) and modified-carbohydrate diet (35% carbohydrate; 30% protein; 35% fat) significantly improved body composition indicators, such as body weight, BMI, waist circumference, and body fat percentage.

However, the improved body composition levels were not significantly different between the low-fat and modified-carbohydrate groups. In addition, significant metabolic improvements were observed in the low-fat diet group (insulin resistance, total and LDL-cholesterol, and C-reactive protein) and the modified-carbohydrate diet group (adiponectin and interleukin-6).

On the other hand, a systemic review of 13 childhood studies compared low-carbohydrate, ad libitum diets with low-fat, energy-restricted diets and reported that the former was more effective for weight loss and blood-lowering lipid levels at six months.

A study shows that among youth aged 6 to 18, a low-carbohydrate diet showed a greater reduction in BMI immediately after dietary intervention than a low-fat diet, even though cardiometabolic benefits from both diets were inconsistent.

Many studies have reported the effectiveness of low-carbohydrate and increased-protein diets on weight reduction, weight maintenance, and improved cardiometabolic risk in obese adults.

Dietary protein is often considered an important nutrient for diet-based weight management because it modulates neuro-endocrine signals related to satiety, thereby having a higher satiating effect than dietary carbohydrates and fat.

Moreover, a high-protein diet showed greater attenuation of a rebound of the relative change in ghrelin over time compared with a high-carbohydrate diet. This was observed in younger children and adults, although another study observed no effects. Sufficient protein intake and physical activity are important for forming body composition, particularly FFM.

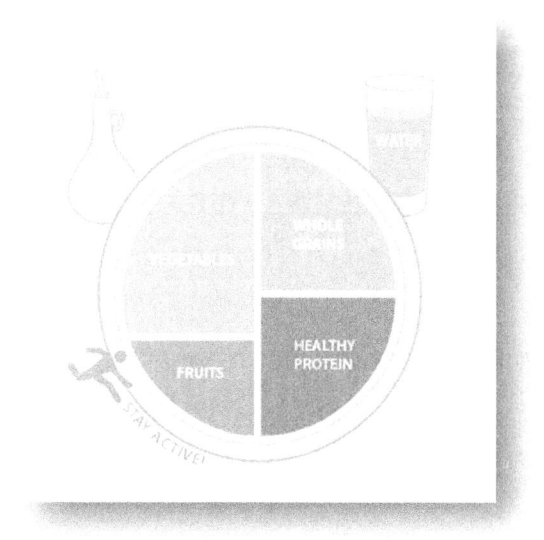

Protein intake was significantly associated with BMI and FFM in young adults in their 20s, increased FFM in children and adolescents, and the maintenance of FFM in elderly people. High-protein diets exceeding 25% of total energy intake or as protein intake ranging from 0.8 g/kg body weight (recommend dietary allowance, RDA) to 1.2–1.6 g/kg (up to double RDA values) in adults improve body composition by preserving lean mass and reducing BFM, especially when combined with training.

In addition, protein intake in the 2.3–3.1 g/kg FFM range was appropriate for lean, resistance-trained athletes in hypocaloric conditions in adults.

In addition to macronutrients, teenagers also need vitamins, minerals, and other micronutrients in their diet to stay healthy. However, the quality and quantity of the macronutrients they consume is especially important.

Chapter 4

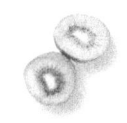

Planning Healthy Meals for Teenagers

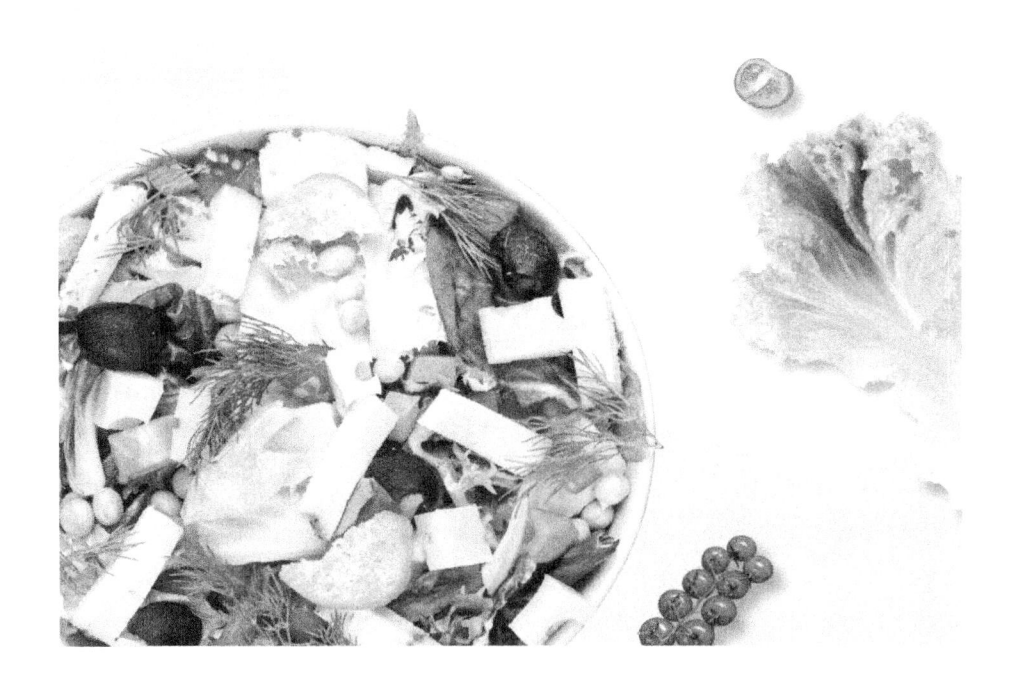

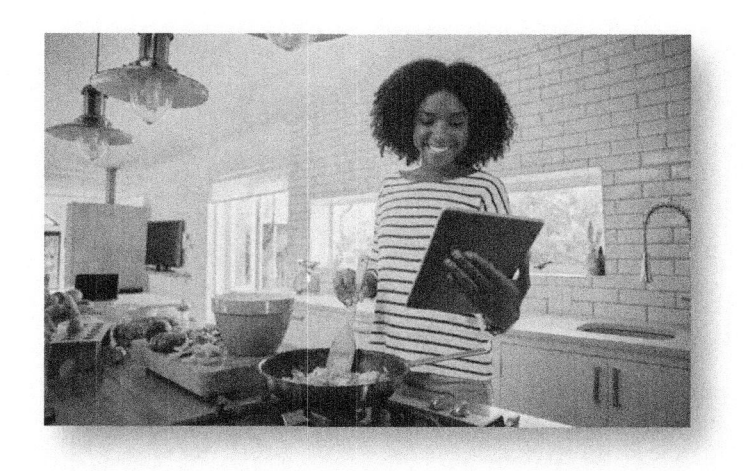

Planning healthy meals for teenagers can be a daunting task. Many teens are picky and may not be interested in eating healthy foods. As a parent or guardian, it is important to provide healthy options for teenagers, as their dietary habits will carry on into adulthood.

This chapter will discuss the importance of planning healthy meals for teenagers, provide tips on how to accommodate picky eaters, and discuss how to create balanced meals.

Additionally, this chapter will provide advice on how to help teenagers become more independent in their meal planning.

By the end of this chapter, the knowledge and skills needed to create healthy meals for teenagers will be crystal clear.

4.1 What is the definition of a healthy meal?

A healthy meal is one that is nutritionally balanced and comprises a variety of foods from different food groups. Balance is key to helping maintain a healthy weight and having the best chance to stay healthy.

It should include a mix of protein, healthy fats, complex carbohydrates, and a variety of vitamins and minerals.

A healthy meal should also be low in sugar, salt, and saturated fat and in appropriate portions to promote a healthy weight.

Protein is important for building and maintaining muscles and other body tissues, and protein sources in a healthy meal include fish, lean meats, poultry, eggs, legumes, nuts, and seeds.

Healthy fats such as olive oil, avocados, and nuts are important for maintaining energy levels and providing essential fatty acids.

Complex carbohydrates are important for providing energy and nutrition, and these can come from whole grains, fruits, and vegetables.

A healthy meal should include a variety of fruits and vegetables, which provide vitamins and minerals, as well as dietary fiber. These foods can be eaten raw, cooked, or in a variety of dishes. Fruits and vegetables also provide antioxidants, which can help protect against disease.

Finally, a healthy meal should be in appropriate portion sizes. Eating too much or too little of any food can lead to weight gain and health problems in the long term. It is important to be mindful of portion sizes when planning meals.

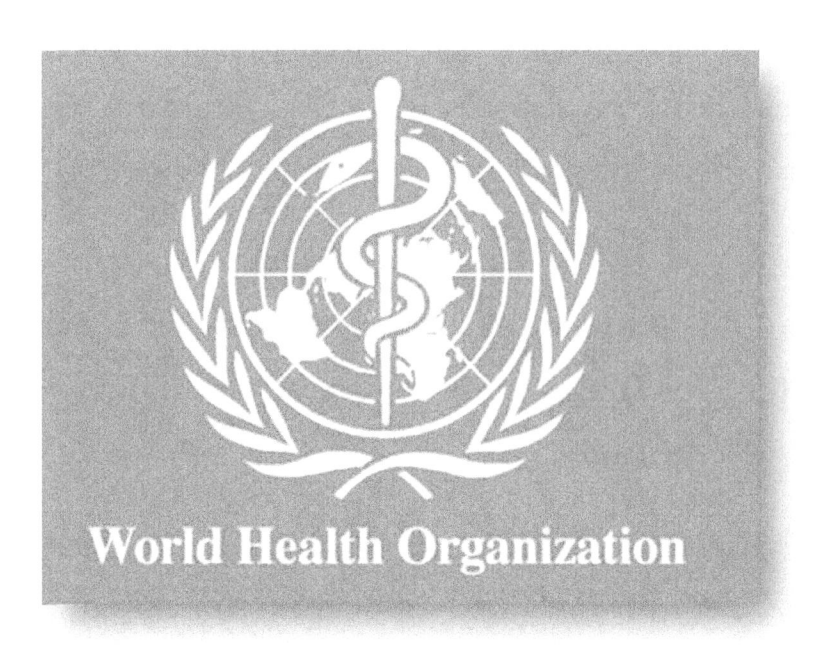

The WHO (the World Health Organization) has given recommendations in 5 points that summarize the basis of nutrition

- Eat roughly the same number of calories that your body uses. Healthy body weight = "calories in"-"calories out."
- Eat a lot of plant foods: vegetables, legumes, whole grains, fruits, and nuts.
- Limit your intake of fats, and prefer healthier unsaturated fats to saturated fats and trans fats.
- Limit your intake of granulated sugar, ideally less than 10g/day.

- Limit salt/sodium consumption from all sources.

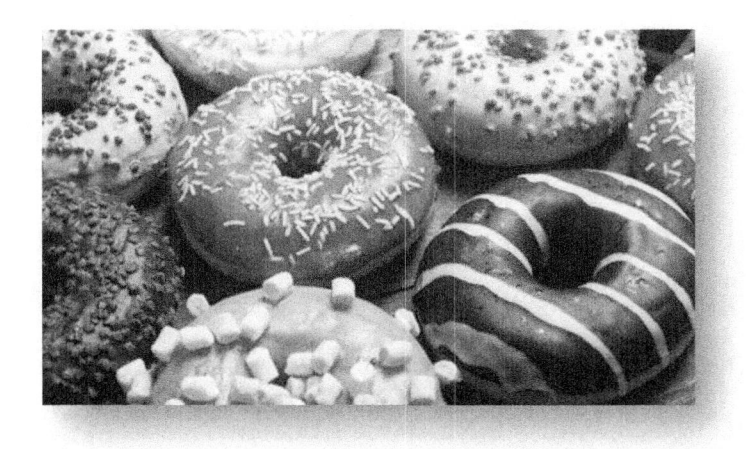

A balanced diet is a pleasure.

Pleasure and variety are important in a balanced diet. Fatty and sweet foods are usually the most delicious and can be part of a balanced diet if eaten in moderation. A balanced diet should bring teens their body needs no more or less, but it must not be strictly followed daily; equilibrium can be achieved over several days.

A balanced diet is for everybody.

At all stages and conditions of life,

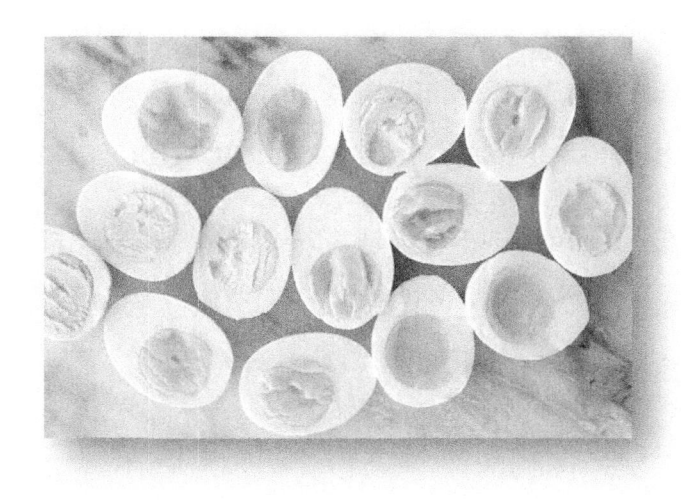

everyone needs a balanced diet that can be adapted while following the same principles, for example:

Teenagers need more protein and calcium for growth, maintenance, or repair. Think of eggs, fish, white meat, legumes, and dairy products.

Students and families might find eating lots of fresh vegetables and fruits expensive and practically difficult. Think of tinned or frozen fruits and vegetables that are cheap and nutritionally as good as fresh ones.

Did you know that tinned sardines are a good source of calcium? They are cheap and also bring proteins and omega-3 fatty acids.

In conclusion, a healthy meal should be nutritionally balanced and include a variety of foods from different food groups. It should be low in sugar, salt, and saturated fat and in appropriate portions. Eating a variety of fruits and vegetables is also important for providing vitamins and minerals, as well as dietary fiber and antioxidants.

By incorporating these components into a teenager's meal, you can ensure that they eat a healthy, balanced diet.

4.2 Learn the benefits of eating healthy.

Eating healthy can boost energy levels and improve concentration, helping teenagers stay focused and perform better in school. Healthy eating can help teens maintain a positive body image and manage stress. Eating healthy is a great way for teenagers to set the foundation for a lifetime of healthy habits. Let's picture some benefits of healthy eating for teens. Below we have mentioned some of the benefits:

Keeps skin, teeth, and eyes healthy

Healthy eating for teenagers is important for keeping their skin, teeth, and eyes healthy. Eating a balanced diet with plenty of fruits and vegetables can provide the body with essential vitamins and minerals, which can help keep the skin, teeth, and eyes healthy. Food such as citrus fruits, leafy greens, lean proteins, and dairy products can all help keep the skin looking and feeling its best.

Calcium-rich foods, such as yogurt and cheese, can help strengthen the teeth and bones.

Additionally, consuming foods rich in vitamin A and beta-carotene can help protect the eyes from age-related degeneration and keep them healthy.

Supports muscles

Healthy eating help teenagers in supporting muscles by providing the body with the right nutrients, minerals, and vitamins essential for muscle growth and development.

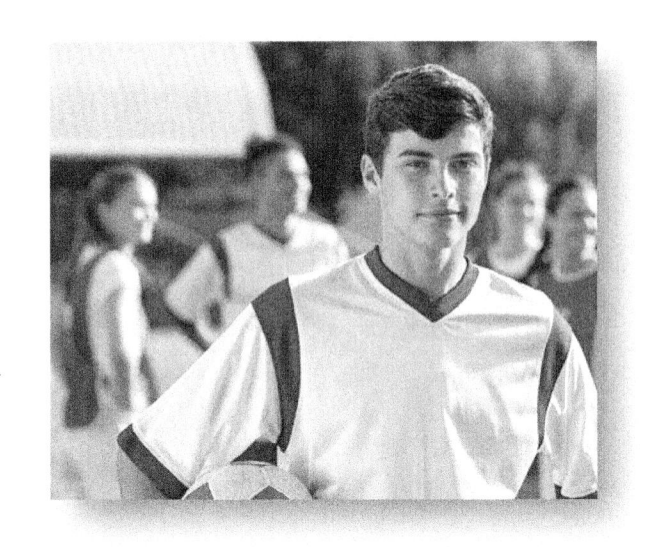

Teenagers eating a balanced diet rich in lean proteins, fruits and vegetables, and healthy fats can help build and maintain muscle mass.

Additionally, consuming adequate amounts of carbohydrates can help support muscle growth and provide the body with energy for physical activities.

Teens regularly eating throughout the day, including small snacks between meals, can also ensure the body gets the nutrients it needs to support muscle development.

Helps achieve and maintain a healthy weight

It helps teens achieve and maintain a healthy weight by focusing on nutrient-dense, low-calorie foods rich in vitamins, minerals, and antioxidants.

Eating various fruits, vegetables, lean proteins, and whole grains provides the nutrients needed for optimal health while avoiding processed foods and beverages high in added sugars, saturated fat, and sodium. Additionally, making mindful, portion-controlled food choices help teens prevent overeating and monitor caloric intake.

These healthy eating habits can help them reach and sustain a healthy weight.

Strengthens bones

Teens eating a diet rich in calcium, Vitamin D, and other minerals help build and maintain strong bones.

Eating foods high in protein, magnesium, and phosphorus also helps keep bones strong and healthy. Eating a variety of healthy foods like fruits, vegetables, and whole grains can provide the body with the vitamins and minerals it needs for bone health.

Additionally, regular exercise can help strengthen bones and muscles and can help prevent bone loss. Eating healthy is important for the overall health of teenagers and can help them maintain strong bones.

Supports brain development

Healthy eating plays an important role in the development of teens' brains. Eating various nutrient-rich foods helps fuel the brain and support its development.

Healthy fats, such as those in nuts, avocados, and fish, are also important for brain development. Eating a balanced diet that includes adequate amounts of vitamins and minerals helps ensure the brain has access to the nutrients it needs to grow and function.

Additionally, healthy eating habits can help to promote a positive attitude and good decision-making skills.

Studies have shown that children who eat a balanced diet are more likely to excel in school and perform well on tests. Eating healthy can help set a strong teen foundation for lifelong health.

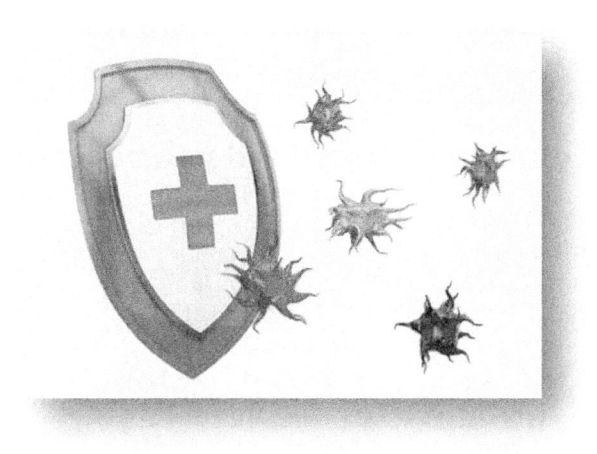

Boosts immunity

It helps teenagers to boost their immunity by providing the body with essential nutrients and vitamins. Eating a variety of nutritious foods can help the body to fight off infections and viruses, as well as protect against chronic diseases.

Eating various foods can also give the body more vitamins and minerals to stay healthy.

Additionally, avoiding processed and sugary foods can help prevent the body from becoming overloaded with unhealthy substances, leading to a weakened immune system. Eating healthy and avoiding processed foods can help boost the body's natural defenses and protect it from disease.

Helps the digestive system function

It helps teens' digestive system function by providing the body with the necessary nutrients and energy to break down and absorb food.

Eating healthy helps to keep the digestive system running smoothly by promoting regular bowel movements and reducing the risk of constipation, acid reflux, and other digestive disorders.

Finally, healthy eating helps reduce inflammation, which can lead to various digestive issues.

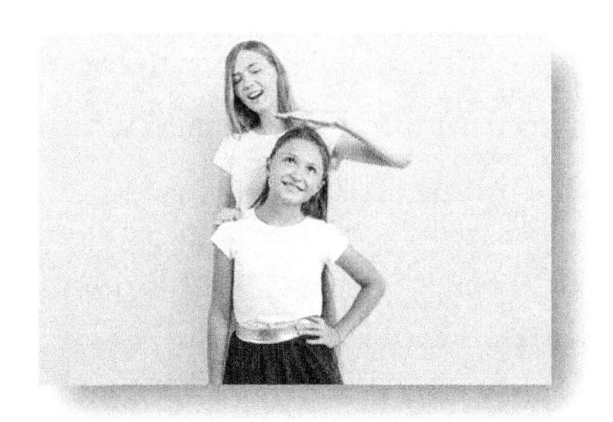

Supports healthy growth

Eating healthy helps to support healthy growth in teenagers and adults alike. Eating a balanced diet low in saturated fat and added sugar can also help reduce the risk of obesity and other chronic diseases. Eating a wide variety of foods can also ensure they get all the necessary vitamins and minerals that their body needs.

4.3 Planning healthy meals for teenagers.

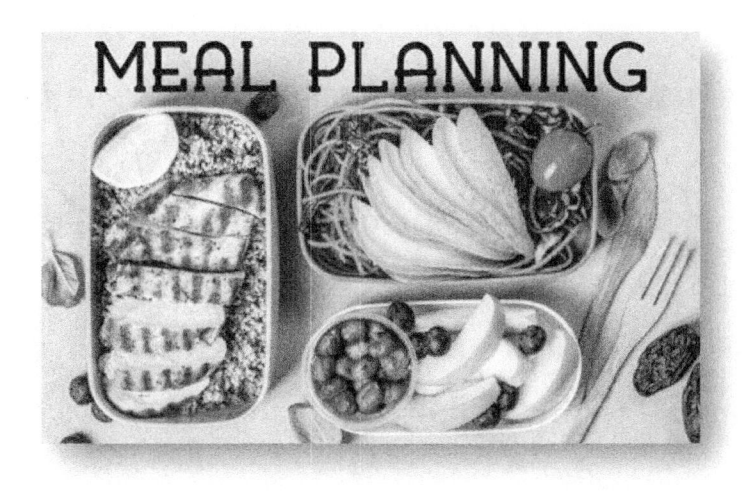

Planning healthy meals for teenagers can be a challenge. Teenagers often have busy schedules and little time for cooking, so meal planning is a great way to ensure they eat nutritious foods. Here are some tips for planning healthy meals for teenagers:

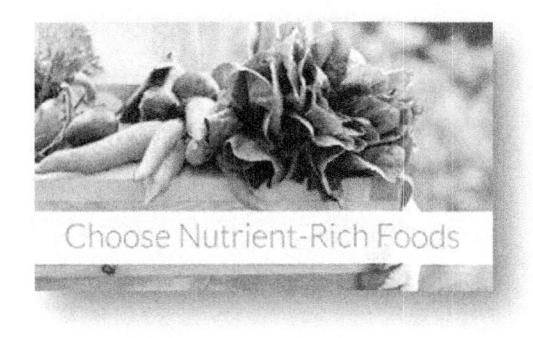

Focus on nutrient-rich foods: When eating healthy, it is important to focus on nutrient-rich foods that provide teenagers with the optimum amount of vitamins, minerals, and other essential nutrients. Eating nutrient-rich foods can help to maintain a healthy weight, reduce the risk of chronic disease, and improve overall health.

In addition to focusing on nutrient-rich foods, limiting the amount of processed and sugary foods teens consume is important. Processed foods often contain added sugars and unhealthy fats and are typically low in essential nutrients. Sugary foods can provide a quick energy boost, but this boost is often followed by an energy crash and can lead to weight gain.

Teenagers should make sure that they drink plenty of water throughout the day to help keep their body hydrated and energized. Water is also important for helping the body to absorb essential vitamins and minerals and for aiding in digestion.

By focusing on nutrient-rich foods, teens can make sure that they are getting the optimum amount of vitamins and minerals that their body needs to stay healthy and energized.

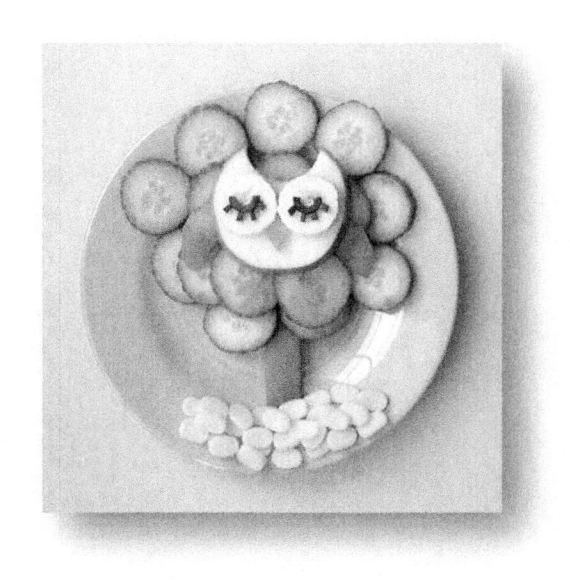

Get creative with snacks: Snacks are an important part of a healthy diet for teenagers. Look for healthy snacks such as:

1. Make a homemade trail mix with your teen's favorite nuts, dried fruit, and seeds.

2. Create a parfait with layers of yogurt, granola, and fresh fruit.

3. Add a snack plate with cheese, crackers, and cured meats.

4. Dried vegetable chips with a garlic-yogurt dip.

5. Fruit kebabs with yogurt dip.

6. Baked sweet potato fries.

7. Mini quiches with an assortment of fillings.

8. Popcorn balls with different flavors of melted chocolate.

9. Roasted chickpeas with spices.

10. Nut and seed bars with honey and dried fruit.

Let teens be involved: It is important to involve them in meal planning to help them develop healthy eating habits and understand how to prepare nutritious meals.

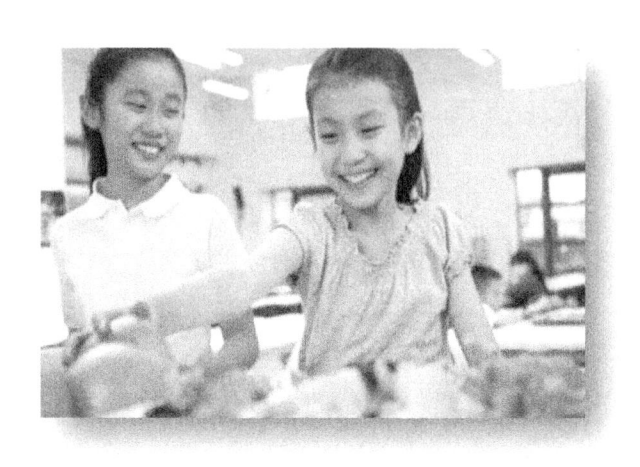

Teens need to learn how to make smart food choices and how to plan meals that will provide them with the nutrients they need for growth and development.

When planning meals, teens can learn to take responsibility for their nutrition. This includes learning how to shop for healthy foods on a budget, understanding the importance of eating a balanced diet, and gaining skills in meal preparation.

Meal planning also teaches teens how to read nutrition labels and make healthy substitutions, so they can make informed decisions about what they eat.

Involving teens in meal planning can also help foster healthy family relationships. Planning meals together allows teens to contribute to the family and develop their sense of autonomy. It also allows parents to provide guidance and instruction on healthy eating habits and cooking techniques.

Additionally, involving teens in meal planning can help promote creativity and experimentation in the kitchen. Teens can take the lead in creating recipes and exploring new flavors. This can help them develop a healthy relationship with food and an appreciation for the culinary arts.

Involvement in meal planning can be a fun and rewarding experience for teens. It can also help them develop important life skills that will benefit them.

Eat together: Eating meals together is a great way to bond and teach teens about healthy eating habits. Try to have family meals at least a few times a week. Eating together is one of the oldest traditions in human history.

It is a time for friends and family to come together, enjoy a meal, and talk about their day, dreams, and lives.

Eating together is a way to bond and create positive relationships. Eating together can

- Provide a sense of unity, as everyone shares in the experience of a meal.
- Help to promote communication and understanding between people.
- Help to reduce stress and build connections between individuals.
- Help to create a healthy lifestyle.
- Make healthier food choices, as they are more conscious of what they eat.
- Encourages people to slow down and savor their meals, aiding in digestion and helping to reduce overeating.
- Be a great way to teach children the importance of healthy eating habits.
- Strengthen relationships, promote healthy eating habits, and create a sense of unity.

It's a time to share stories, offer advice, and listen to one another.

In addition to the emotional benefits of eating together, there are also some physical benefits. By sitting down together, parents can model healthy eating habits and discuss the nutritional value of their food. This helps children to make healthier choices in their own lives.

In today's world, it is easy to forget the importance of eating together. We are often too busy with our own lives to take the time to sit down and enjoy a meal with those we care about.

However, taking the time to eat together can incredibly impact our lives. Eating together can

By following these tips, you can help ensure that teenagers eat nutritious foods and develop healthy eating habits.

4.4 Encouraging healthy eating habits for teens.

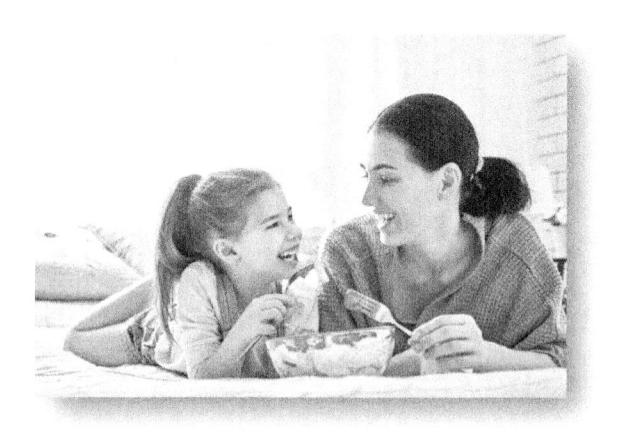

About one in three children in the United States is overweight or obese, and sadly an overweight child has a 70 to 80 percent chance of staying overweight as an adult.

As a result, it's important to establish good nutrition habits for your children. Parents must encourage their teens to develop healthy eating habits, which will help them stay healthy and active in their teenage years and beyond.

While you certainly can't control everything your teen eats, you can role model healthy eating, discuss what makes up a nutritious diet, and prepare healthy meals for your family. Here are some steps to take:

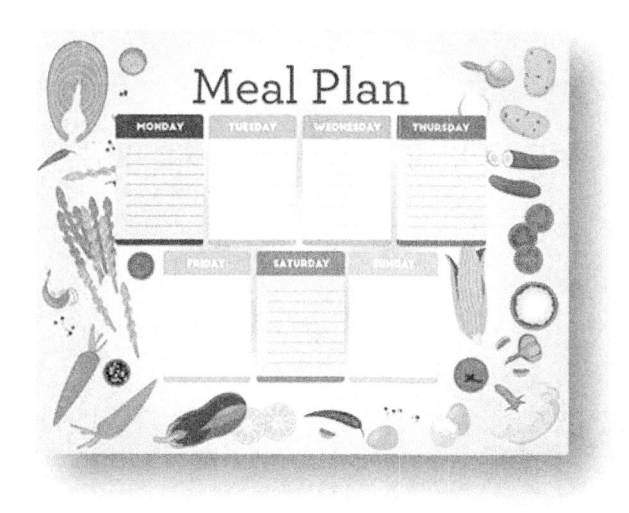

One way to encourage healthy eating habits for teens is to have them plan their meals. Have them plan a week's worth of meals and snacks, and then ensure they have the ingredients to prepare them. This will help them to focus on eating healthier foods.

Another way to encourage healthy eating habits is to provide healthy snacks and meals. Offer healthy teen snacks.

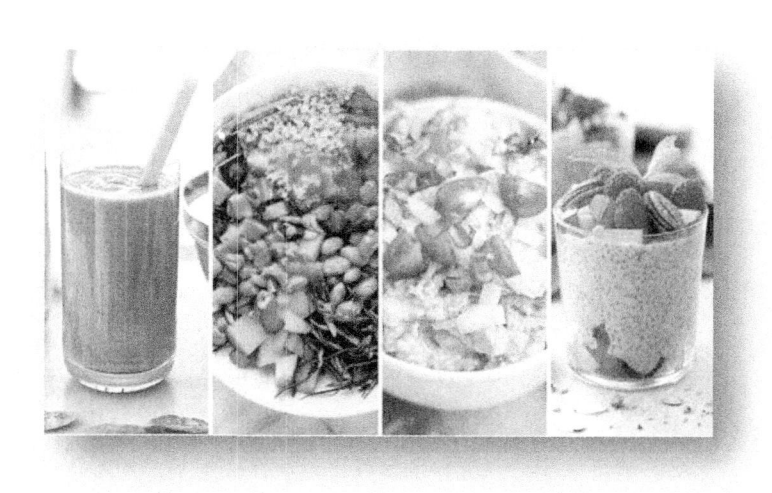

Make sure to include a variety of foods to give your teen a balanced diet. For meals, serving a combination of fruits, vegetables, proteins, and whole grains is a good idea.

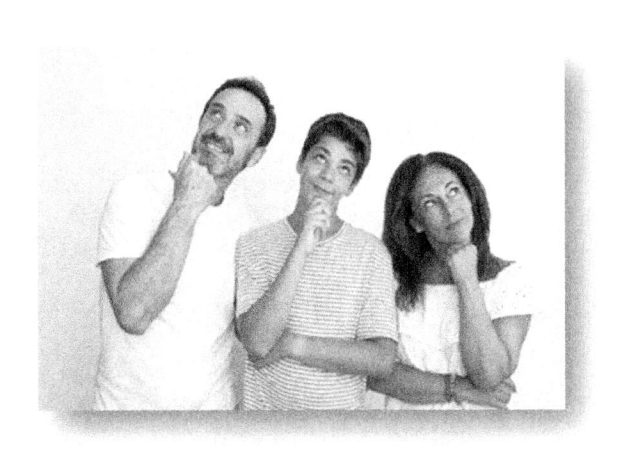

Final Thoughts

Your teen closely observes your lifestyle, eating habits, and attitudes about appearance and weight, even if it doesn't seem like it, so you must be a good role model.

Do not use food as a reward, punishment, or a way to manage your emotions. Do not try to lose or gain weight dramatically or use fad diets, but rather work towards a healthy weight by eating a well-balanced, nutritious, and healthy diet.

"Everything in moderation" is far more positive to share with your children than messages about food exclusion and restrictive dieting.

Chapter 5

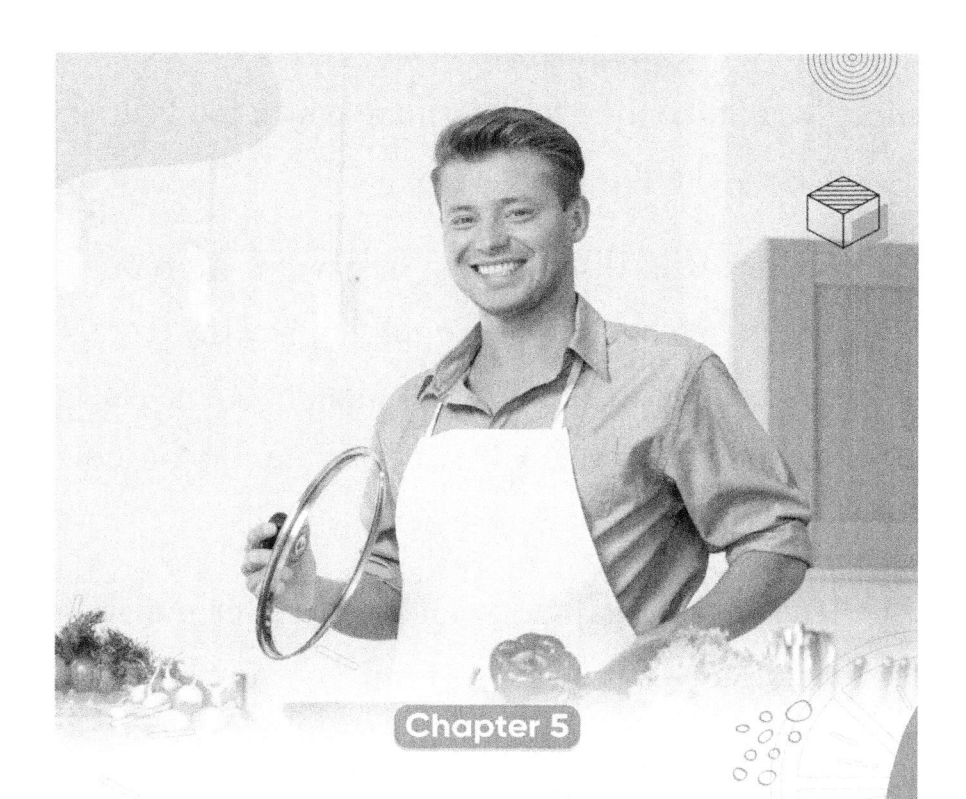

Making Healthy Choices at Home

Shopping for healthy food can be a challenging task. With the multitude of options available in grocery stores and online, it can take time to determine which foods are best for teenagers' health.

This chapter will discuss the basics of shopping for healthy foods. We will cover identifying healthy foods and making smart food choices to ensure they get the nutrition they need. We will also provide tips on how to save money while shopping for healthy foods.

By the end of this chapter, you should better understand how to shop for healthy foods to make informed choices that will benefit a teen's overall health.

5.1 Learn a few tips for shopping for healthy foods.

Did you know that the average supermarket carries 38,718 products? No wonder navigating the aisles can feel overwhelming!

When you add the temptation to grab less-than-healthy choices for teens, a grocery store trip seems more like a battle than an opportunity to fill your cart – and your body – with wholesome, good-for-you foods.

But with these simple shopping strategies, you can skip the stress and leave the market with bags full of healthy options.

Go With a Plan

Before heading to the store, think about the meals you will prepare over the coming week and list the ingredients. You can save time in the store by grouping the ingredients on your list by department or aisle (produce, dairy, frozen, etc.), so you can stock up more efficiently.

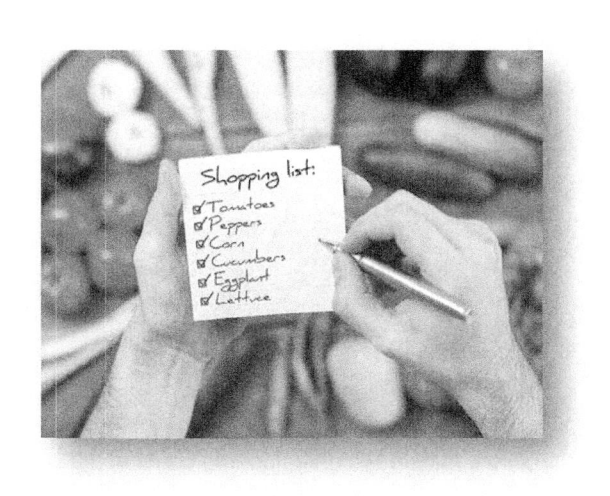

Stick to your list to avoid wandering through the store and buying items you don't need or aren't the healthiest.

Have a Snack First

It may sound silly, but it works – eating a little before you shop helps you avoid the temptation of buying junk food or filling your cart with more than you need.

Protein gives a snack staying power, so try dipping apple slices or celery sticks in peanut butter or pair whole grain crackers with a small portion of hard cheese like parmesan, low-fat swiss, or low-fat cheddar before you head to the store.

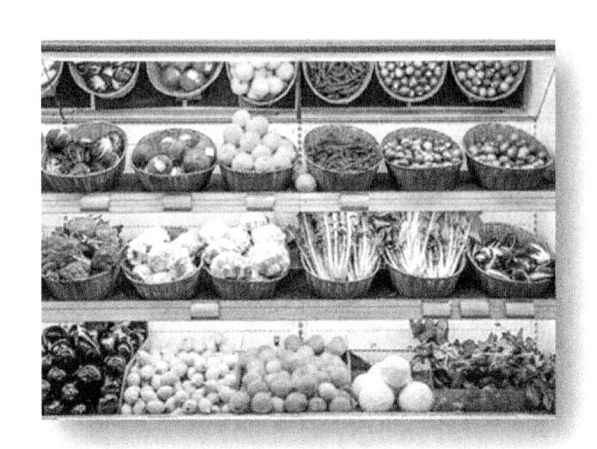

Shop the Perimeter

The outer aisles of the grocery store are where you can find the freshest, least processed foods – fruits, vegetables, meats, fish, dairy, and bread. Aim to get most of your food there.

Choose Seasonal Produce

Fruits and vegetables in season are usually more nutritious, abundant, tasty, and inexpensive than those out of season

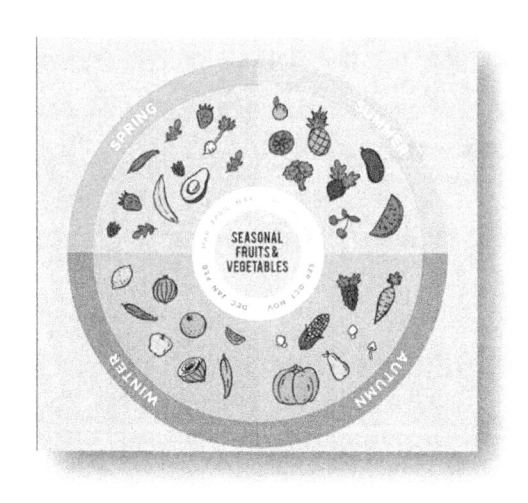

– making them a great choice all around!

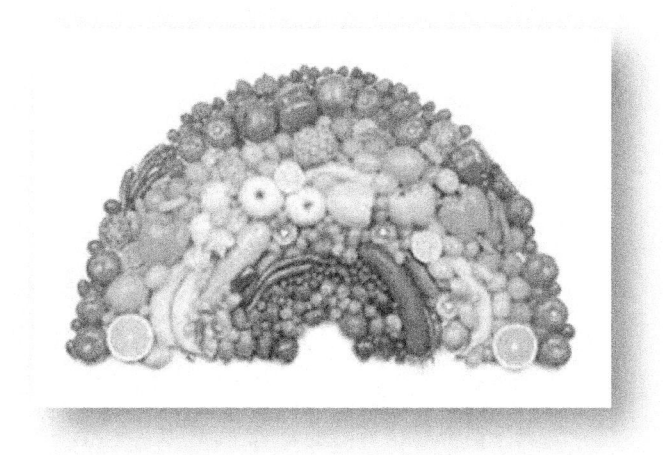

Buy the Rainbow

The USDA recommends filling half our plates with colorful fruits and vegetables at mealtimes since it helps with calorie management and ensures the consumption of various nutrients. Your cart should reflect this suggestion. Green is great, but how about a bright red tomato or a beautiful pint of blueberries?

Don't Buy Now If You Don't Want to Be Tempted Later

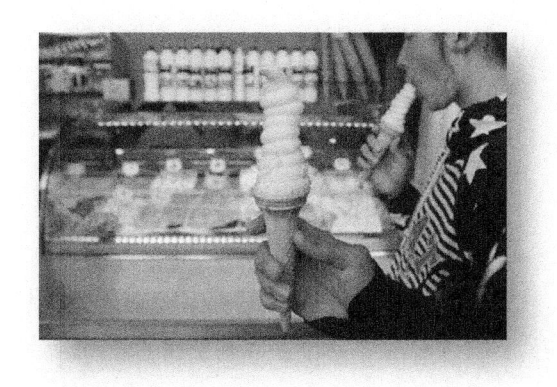

This one sound obvious enough, but it's easy to forget. Think about what foods you tend to overindulge in, and if you can't seem to limit your serving sizes, keep them out of the house and allow yourself to indulge in a sensible portion when you're out instead. After all, isn't enjoying a scoop of your favorite flavor at the local ice cream shop more fun than eating a pint of the rocky road while standing over the sink at home?

Broaden Your Shopping Horizons

Supermarkets are easy to come by, but farmer's markets, food co-ops, and Community Supported Agriculture (CSA) programs are growing in popularity and abundance. They offer fresh, local produce (often organic), and many sell locally sourced meats, dairy products, and bread. Try switching or working some of these options into your shopping plans. Find a farmers' market, co-op, or CSA near you.

5.2 Comparison between the benefits of buying local and organic

Which is best for people and the planet? And how do we make truly healthy food accessible to all?

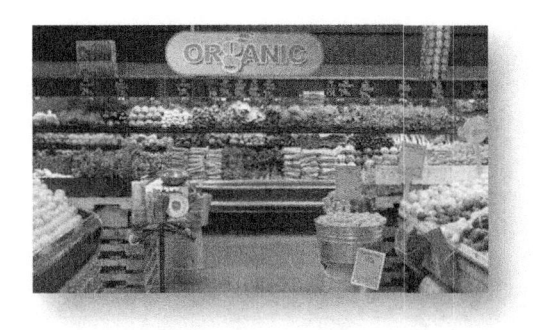

You walk into the grocery store, wanting to buy some Granny Smith apples for a pie you're planning to bake. There are two types—organic apples from across the country or from a local farm that uses chemical pesticides and herbicides. Which do you choose?

The climate-change benefits of organic food are almost negated when that food has traveled a long distance from farm to plate. In response, the "locavore" movement—or people dedicated to buying much of their food in season from local farms—enjoyed a resurgence in popularity, casting doubts on the wisdom of always buying organic.

The Case for Organic

Organic farming sequesters more carbon in the soil than conventional chemical farming. And it uses no chemical inputs, which must be trucked in from long distances and spread across fields using fossil fuel-powered machinery.

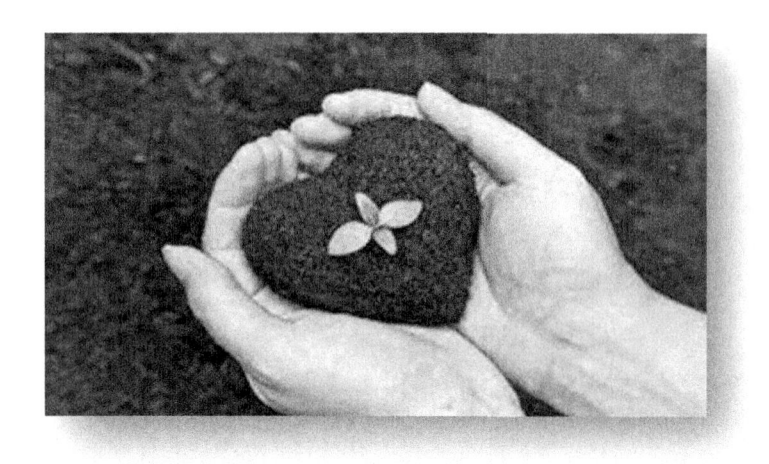

Organically farmed soil sequesters nearly 30 percent more carbon than chemically farmed soil.

If all 3.5 billion acres of farmland on the planet were farmed organically, the soil would sequester nearly 40 percent of the world's carbon dioxide (CO_2) emissions, and converting all 434 million acres of US farmland to organic would sequester nearly 1.6 billion tons of CO_2 per year, the equivalent of taking 800,000 cars off the road annually.

In addition, farming chemicals must be transported by air, train, or truck from the factory to the farm, which may be a long distance—further adding to the climate impact of conventional farms.

Farm Chemicals Poison our Bodies

An extensive body of evidence demonstrates that pesticides harm workers, damage the environment, and demonstrate toxicity to laboratory animals. When you can't find out how a local food was grown, recommend choosing organic, which guarantees that no pesticides or chemical fertilizers were used to grow it.

Organic Could Feed the World

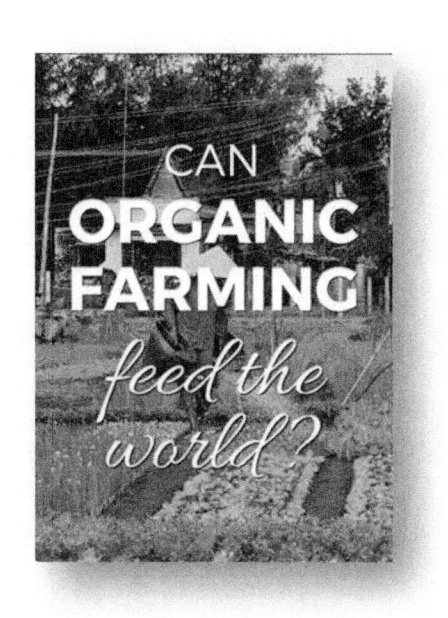

One of the main arguments against a worldwide shift to organics is the allegation that organic farms can't possibly feed the world. However, yield rates for different types of food grown organically and non-organically. It found that "organic methods could produce enough food on a global per capita basis to sustain the current population, and potentially even a larger population, without increasing the agricultural land base." Part of the reason is that the average agricultural yield worldwide is much lower than that of state-of-the-art organic farming.

Organic Just May Be Healthier

Organic food is nutritionally similar to conventional food.

Organics came out significantly better in three of the 13 nutrient categories; Organics contained more beneficial phosphorus and titratable acids. And conventional foods contain more nitrogen, which may be linked to cancer—the health effects of additives and pesticide residues in conventional produce.

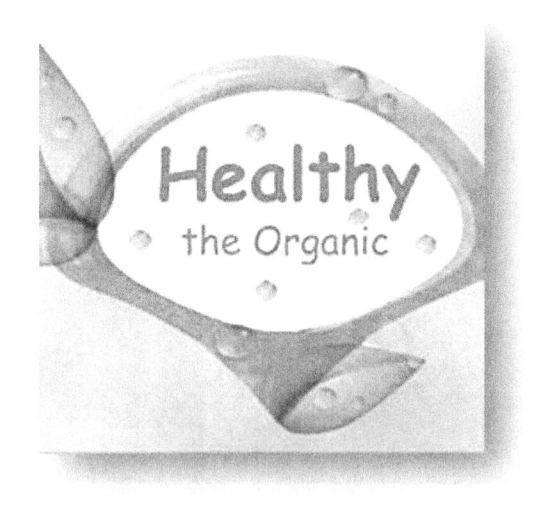

Some types of organic produce have been found to contain "significantly more" cancer-fighting antioxidants than conventional produce.

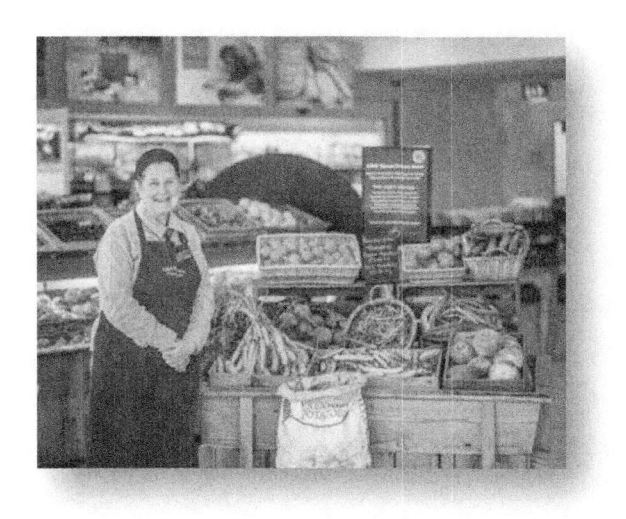

Where Local Fits In

"There comes a time when we all have to agree—or agree to agree on major points. There's enough evidence to know that embracing organic is right."

Organic standards are strong enough that shoppers can trust the label regarding toxins.

It's not perfect. The reality is that certified organic food can come from big agribusinesses, some of which have many of the problems of industrial agriculture—from the loss of biodiversity to raising animals in crowded fields. This may be organic, but it is not sustainable. To have a truly restorative and healthy food system, it must be organic and local.

However, because of the seriousness of the toxic chemical burden and climate footprint of conventional agriculture.

While organic standards are good, we must improve them, "We must work together to create the best definition of what organic means, to include social justice and Fair-Trade standards and humanely raised animals and more."

5.3 Pick up some tips for eating healthy on a budget

Eating healthy when money is tight can be challenging. These tips can help.

A diet with plenty of vegetables, fruits, and lean proteins is important for good health for teens. Healthy eating is key to maintaining blood sugar levels in your target range. But the cost of nutritious foods can quickly add up.

Eating on a budget doesn't mean you have to sacrifice nutrition. With some know-how and planning, you can enjoy nutritious foods without breaking the bank.

Following these six tips may surprise you at how much you can stretch your grocery budget.

Plan Your Recipes

Planning let's consider food needs, tastes, and budget. If you know you must stretch your money for the week, meal planning can pay off.

Adapt recipes to fit teens' needs. If they love pasta dishes and follow a low-carb diet, you can search for recipes that use veggie noodles instead of traditional noodles. These are great alternatives to increase their vegetable intake.

Use recipes with common ingredients. Using the same ingredients for multiple meals means they can taste different. Using different herbs and spices can turn common ingredients into meals with different flavors. If teens love chicken, cook one whole chicken and use it for several dishes. You can have chicken and vegetable stir fry one night and chicken fajitas another night.

Find ways to stretch a recipe. You can stretch meals by making dishes that freeze well. Search online for delicious healthy recipes like soups and casseroles that are budget-friendly and easy meals to stretch. For example, make a large batch of vegetable soup or white bean chicken chili that lasts throughout the week, or freeze the leftovers later. You'll also spend less time in the kitchen than if you make a different meal every night.

Planning a weekly menu also increases the chance that your pantry and refrigerator are stocked with healthy ingredients to make balanced meals.

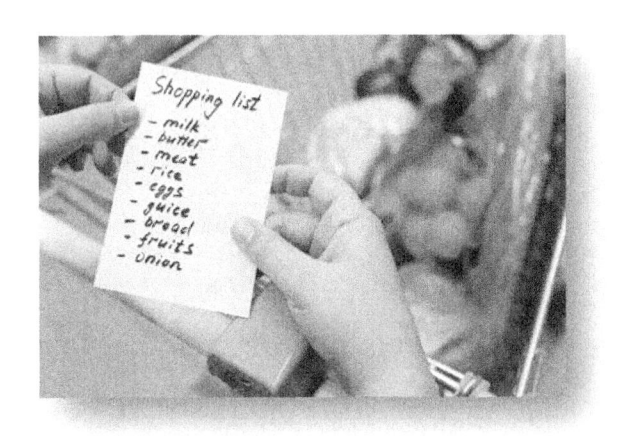

Shop with a List

Once we've planned meals for the week, create a shopping list with the ingredients we need. A shopping list makes shopping easier and faster, which helps us reduce impulse buys and take home only the items we need.

It also helps us avoid extra trips to the grocery store to buy forgotten items. If the shopping list includes nuts, beans, or grains, consider buying in bulk to save money and keep the pantry well-stocked for future meal planning.

Buy Frozen or Canned

Regarding fruits and vegetables, frozen and canned options can be healthy alternatives to fresh produce. What's more, they cost less and last longer. Many frozen veggies and fruits have resealable packaging that allows you to use what you need and store the rest. This way, you can enjoy your favorites even when they aren't in season.

When choosing canned options, selecting those that come in water, not syrup, is best. Be sure to read the label for any added sugar or salt. You'll want to avoid those. And skip frozen options that have added butter or cream sauces. Choose options without sauce or look for packaging that reads "lightly sauced" to avoid extra sugar, salt, and empty calories.

Cut Cost with Coupons

Coupons are a great way to save on your grocery bill, especially if you have your shopping list planned out. You can search for online coupons for the ingredients on your list. With over a billion coupons available each year, you will likely find a coupon that you can use.

If you can't find a coupon for those blueberries on your list but find one for strawberries, consider swapping to save money. Even low-value cents-off coupons can add up. Just by using five 50-cents-off coupons a week, you can save over $100 each year.

Buy Store Brands

Buying generic or store-brand items can save you 20% to 30% on your food bill. Items like canned tomatoes, milk, olive oil, and frozen fruits and vegetables are usually available in a cheaper store-brand version. Just compare the ingredients list and nutrition facts panel to ensure you're not getting a product with added ingredients. Learning which store brands your grocery store carries can help you reduce your total at the cash register.

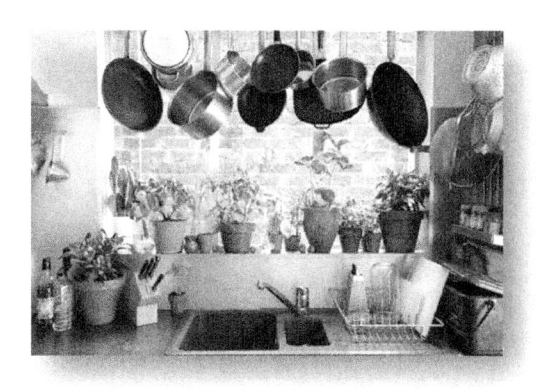

Try Growing a Garden

Growing your fruits and vegetables is a great way to save money, have fresh produce at your fingertips, and make teens eat that. Even if you don't have a garden yard, many fruits, vegetables, and herbs can grow in pots on patios or balconies. A constant supply of fresh produce at home can save you money at the store. You may not be able to grow a "money tree" in your garden, but it'll feel like you did with the extra money you'll be saving.

Chapter 6

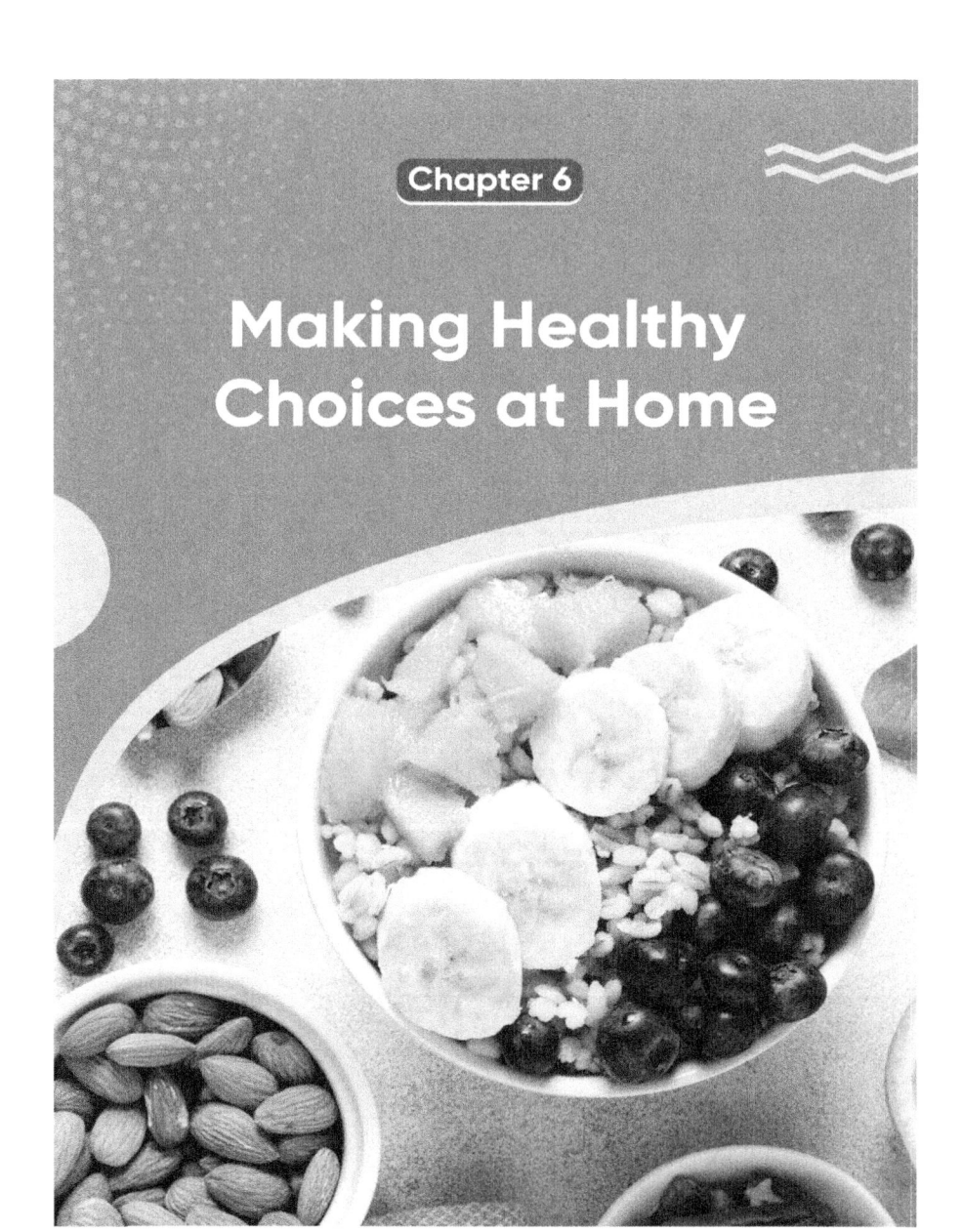

Making Healthy Choices at Home

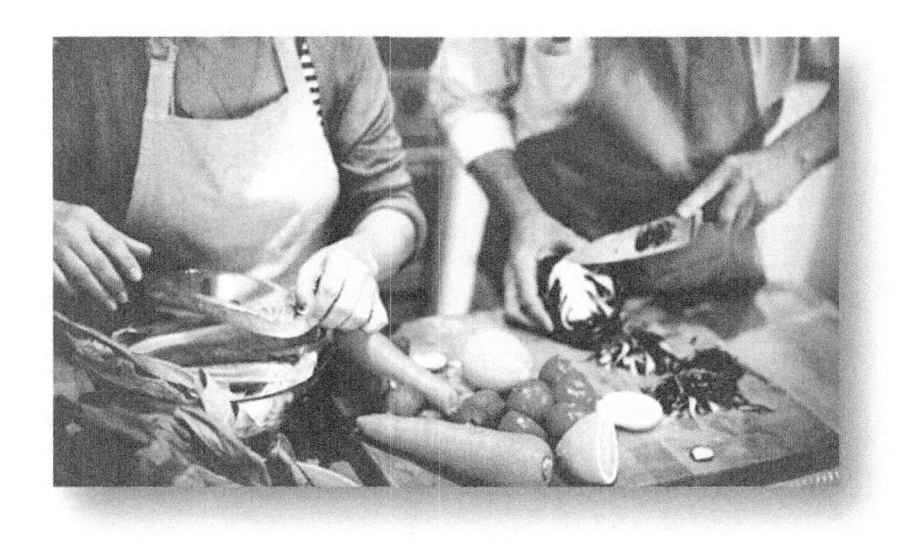

Making healthy choices at home is important to staying healthy and happy as a teenager. Eating healthy, getting enough sleep, and staying active are all key components of healthy choices at home.

In this chapter, we will explore how teens can make the most of their home environment by setting up healthy routines, choosing nutritious foods, and engaging in activities that promote physical and mental well-being. We will also discuss how teens can make healthy choices on their own and with their families and how to manage stress and stay organized. By implementing these tips, teens can create an environment supporting them in pursuing a healthy lifestyle.

6.1 Determine meal planning and preparation

Figuring out what to eat daily can be stressful, especially when juggling a busy schedule that includes work, family, and social obligations. Often, people scrape together last-minute meals, throw them in the hat, and order food delivery. Rest assured. Meal planning is a better way to feed teens and families. This approach ensures that you're never left wondering what's for dinner.

What Is Meal Planning?

Meal planning is building a weekly menu to suit your nutritional needs best. "It can take the guesswork out of dinnertime, help you to stick to a budget, and help keep your nutrition goals on track,"

Some people follow a meal plan with a specific outcome, plan to stick to a food budget or map out meals for an entire family.

There are different types of meal plans.

People who aren't trying to manage a health condition typically make their meal plans by selecting healthy recipes that their families enjoy.

So, here we have something for you.

1. High Protein Meal Plan:

Breakfast: Omelet made with 2 eggs and diced vegetables, 1/2 cup of oatmeal, and a side of fruit

Lunch: Grilled chicken breast, 1 cup of brown rice, and a side salad

Snack: Protein shake and a handful of nuts

Dinner: Salmon filet, 1 cup of quinoa, and steamed vegetables

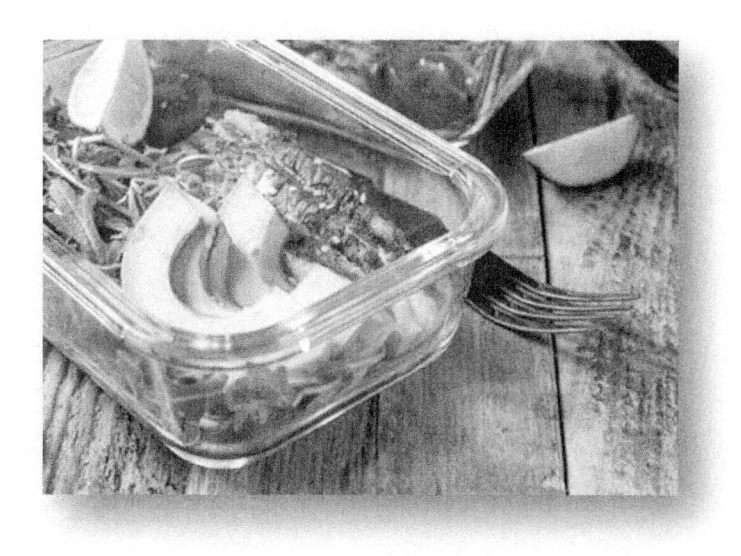

2. Vegetarian Meal Plan:

Breakfast: Scrambled tofu with vegetables, 1/2 cup of oatmeal, and a side of fruit

Lunch: Hummus wrap with vegetables and a side salad

Snack: Smoothie made with greens and nut butter

Dinner: Veggie stir-fry with 1/2 cup of brown rice and a side of steamed broccoli.

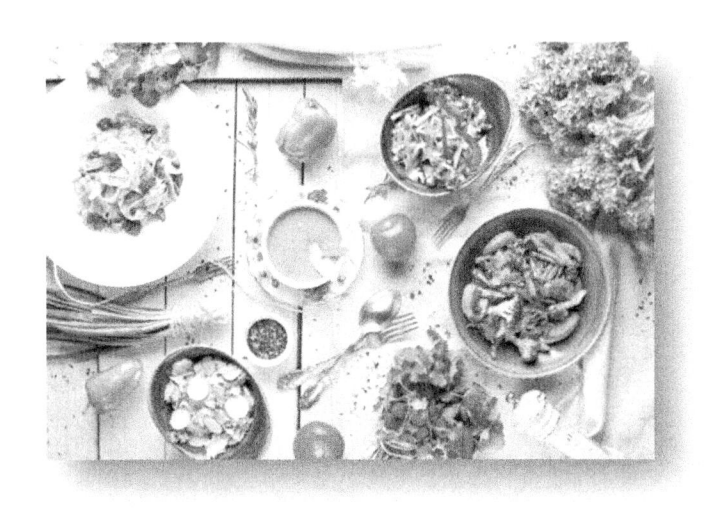

3. Low-Calorie Meal Plan:

Breakfast: Oatmeal with fresh fruit and a sprinkle of cinnamon

Lunch: Garden salad with grilled chicken and a balsamic vinaigrette

Snack: Greek yogurt with fresh berries

Dinner: Grilled fish, roasted vegetables, and a side of quinoa

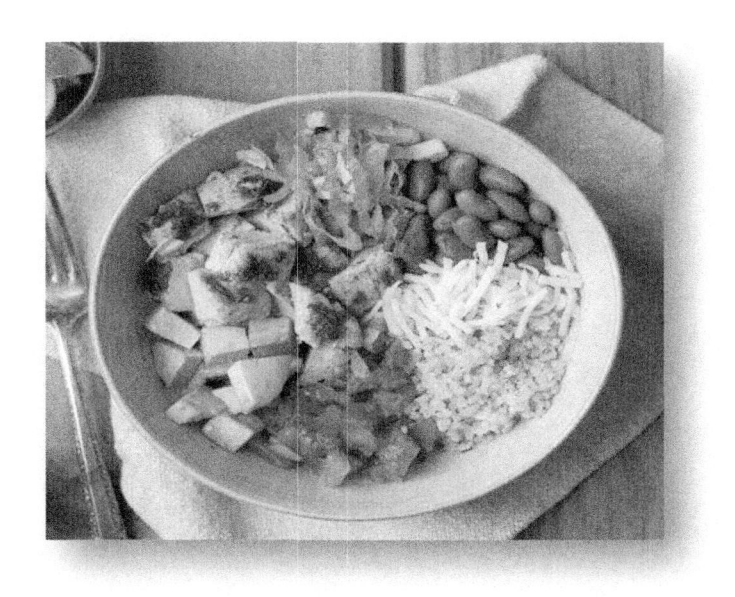

4. Low-Carb Meal Plan:

Breakfast: Egg omelet with diced vegetables, 1/2 avocado, and a side of berries

Lunch: Grilled chicken breast, steamed vegetables, and a side of guacamole

Snack: Hard-boiled egg and a few slices of deli meat

Dinner: Baked salmon, roasted cauliflower, and a side of sautéed spinach.

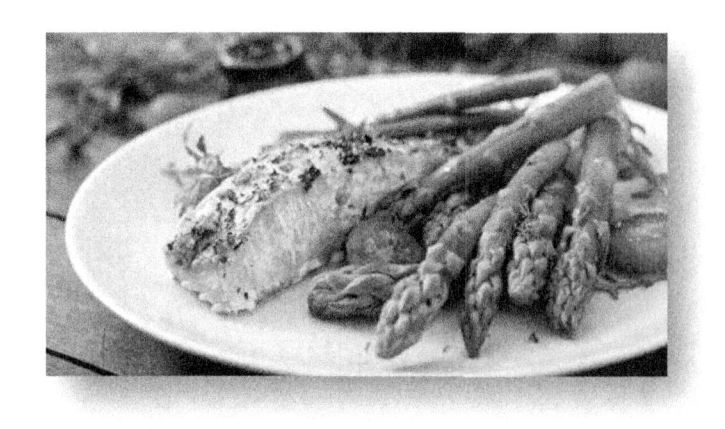

6.2 Pursue limiting processed foods.

Processed foods are an important part of the modern diet, providing convenience and variety. However, they can also be high in unhealthy fats, salt, and sugar, and contain artificial additives and chemicals. To maintain a healthy diet, it is important to limit processed foods, and focus on eating whole, natural foods that are as close to their natural state as possible. Here are some tips for limiting processed foods:

1. Read Food Labels: Whenever possible, read the food label and look for added sugars, unhealthy fats, and artificial additives. If the food contains too much of these, it is best to choose a healthier alternative.

2. Choose Whole Foods: Whole foods are foods that are in their natural state and are not processed.

Examples include fruits, vegetables, whole grains, nuts, and legumes. These foods provide more vitamins, minerals, and fiber than their processed counterparts.

3. Buy Fresh or Frozen Produce: Fresh produce is often more nutritious than canned or processed produce. If fresh produce is not available, frozen produce is a good alternative. Frozen produce is usually picked at its peak freshness and flash-frozen to retain its nutritional content.

4. Limit Processed Meat: Processed meats like bacon, hot dogs, and deli meats are high in saturated fat and salt. It is best to limit these foods and opt for leaner cuts of meat, such as skinless chicken and fish.

5. Avoid Pre-Made Meals: Pre-made meals, such as frozen dinners and microwaveable meals, are usually high in sodium and other unhealthy ingredients. It is best to make meals from scratch with fresh ingredients.

6. Buy Natural Snacks: When it comes to snacks, look for snacks with few ingredients and no added sugars or unhealthy fats. Examples include nuts, seeds, fruits, and vegetables.

7. Cook More at Home: Home-cooked meals are usually healthier than restaurant meals or pre-made meals. They also provide the opportunity to control what ingredients are used and how they are prepared.

These tips can help you limit processed foods and eat a healthier diet. Remember, it is important to choose whole, natural foods whenever possible, and to read food labels carefully. With a bit of planning and preparation, you can create delicious, healthy meals that are good for you and your family.

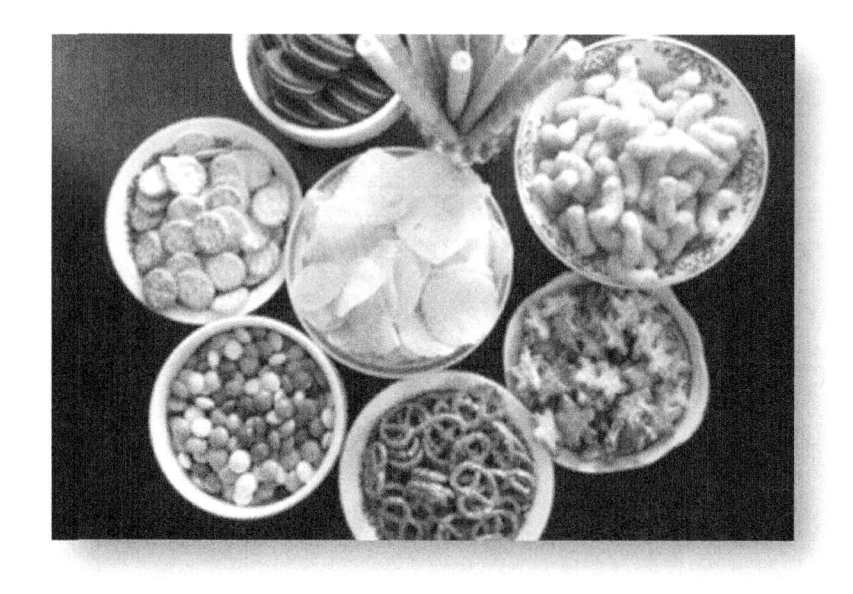

6.3 Why is staying hydrated equally important as healthy eating?

Staying hydrated is just as important as eating healthy for overall health and wellbeing. While healthy eating is widely recognized for its importance in maintaining good health, staying hydrated is also essential for optimal health. Adequate hydration helps with digestion, flushes out toxins and waste, keeps skin looking healthy, and even helps with weight loss.

Water makes up about 60% of the human body and is necessary for many of its processes. It transports nutrients and oxygen to cells, helps regulate body temperature, and is a key component in many bodily functions. Water is also necessary for digestion and helps to flush out toxins and waste. Without proper hydration, the body can't function properly.

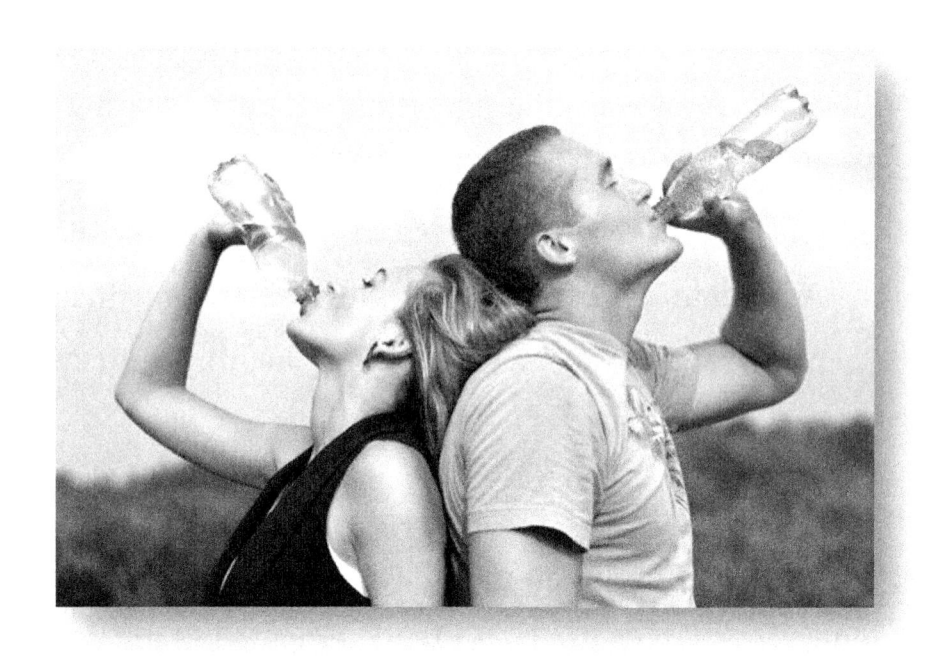

Staying hydrated also helps keep skin looking healthy and vibrant. Water helps to flush out toxins and impurities, which can help to reduce the appearance of wrinkles and other signs of aging. It also helps keep skin moisturized and supple, which can help to reduce skin irritation and dryness.

Adequate hydration can even help with weight loss. Drinking water before meals can help to reduce hunger and make you feel fuller faster. This can help to reduce the amount of food consumed at meals, resulting in fewer calories consumed overall.

Additionally, drinking water can help to increase energy levels, which can help to increase the amount of physical activity in which one engages.

Overall, staying hydrated is just as important as eating healthy for overall health and wellbeing. Adequate hydration helps to flush out toxins and waste, keep skin looking healthy, and even help with weight loss. It is important to ensure that one is getting enough water throughout the day in order to stay healthy and avoid dehydration. In addition to drinking plenty of water, consuming foods with a high water content, such as fruits and vegetables, can also help to increase hydration levels.

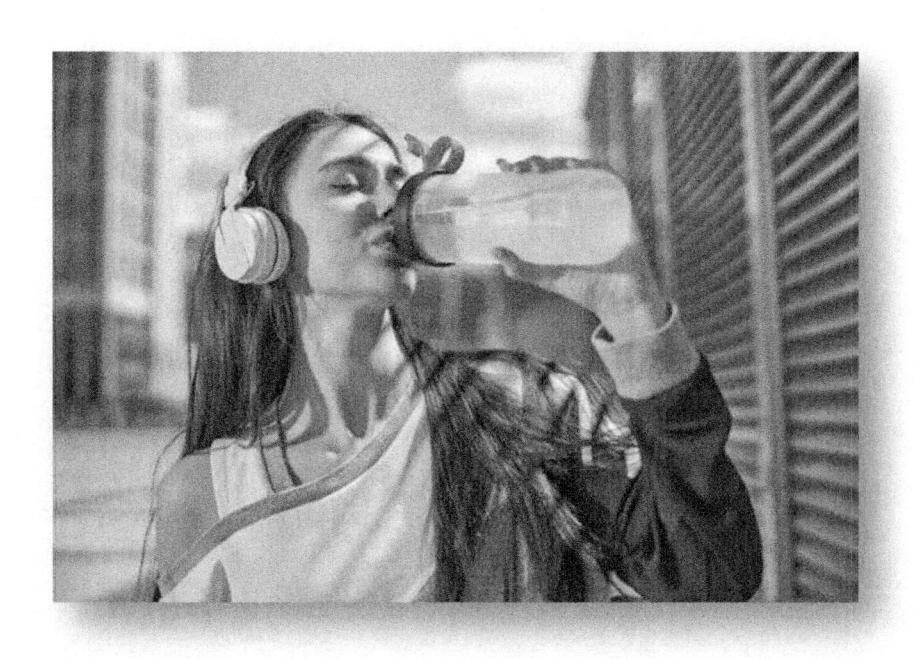

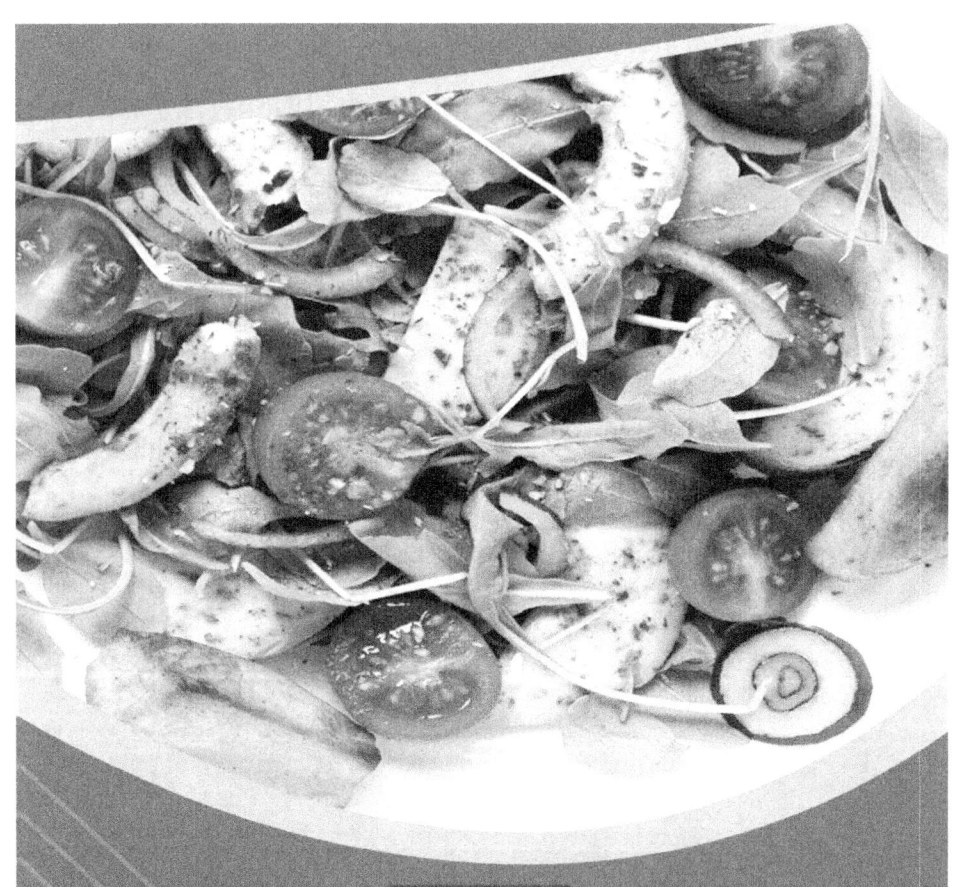

Chapter 7

Strategies
for Eating Healthy While Out

Eating healthy while out can sometimes be a challenge. With the abundance of fast food and processed food options, it can be hard to make healthy choices. However, with the right strategies eating healthy while out can be easier than you think.

This introduction will provide some tips and tricks for maintaining a healthy diet when you're on the go. From planning to making smarter choices at restaurants, these strategies will help you make nutritious decisions when you're out and about.

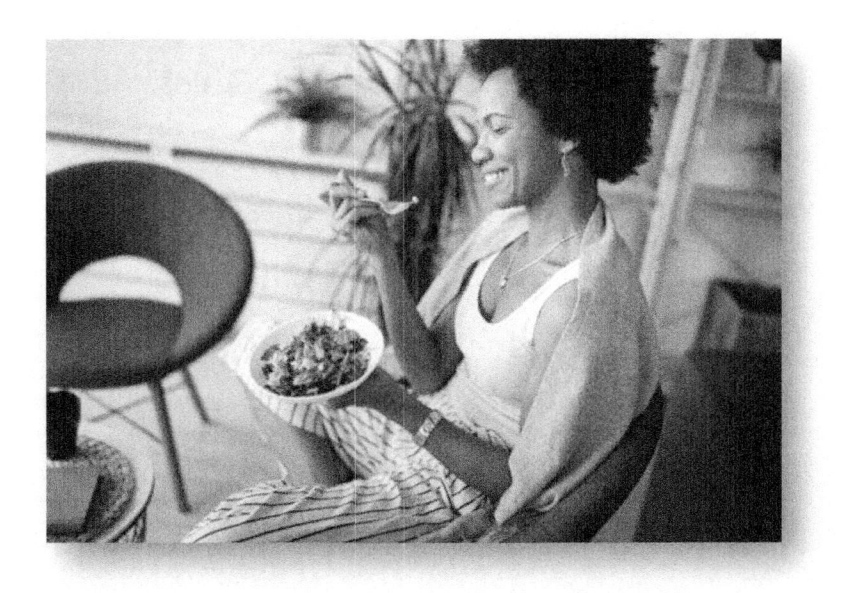

7.1 Learn a few healthy eating out options

Eating out can be a challenge when you are trying to maintain a healthy diet.

Most restaurants have menus full of unhealthy options high in calories, fat, and sodium. But fortunately, with a few strategies and a little knowledge, you can enjoy a meal away from home without compromising your health. Here are a few tips on healthy eating when dining out.

- **Look for grilled options** - Grilled meats and vegetables tend to be much lower in fat and calories than fried or sautéed dishes. Try to avoid dishes that are fried or covered in creamy sauces.
- **Opt for a salad or soup** - Salads are a great option for a healthy starter. Look for salads with lots of leafy greens and colorful vegetables. Soups can also be a nutritious choice. Try to avoid creamy soups, which are often full of fat and calories.
- **Choose lean proteins** - Lean proteins such as chicken, fish, and turkey are much better options than fatty red meats. If possible, ask your server to grill or bake your protein instead of frying it.
- **Watch your portion size** - Many restaurants offer large portions that can be difficult to resist. If you are served a generous portion, ask your server for a to-go box so you can save half of your meal for later.

- **Ask for dressings and sauces on the side** - Dressings and sauces can add a lot of fat and calories to your meal. Ask for them on the side so you can control how much you are eating.
- **Skip the bread basket** - Breads, rolls, and other starchy foods are often high in calories and low in nutritional value. If you want a little something to munch on, ask for a side of vegetables or a piece of fruit instead.
- **Drink water** - Sugary sodas and alcoholic beverages can quickly add up when you are eating out. Stick to water for a healthier option.

With a few simple strategies, you can enjoy eating out without compromising your health. Look for grilled options, choose lean proteins, ask for dressings and sauces on the side, skip the bread basket, and drink water. With a little knowledge and a few healthy choices, you can enjoy a delicious and nutritious meal away from home.

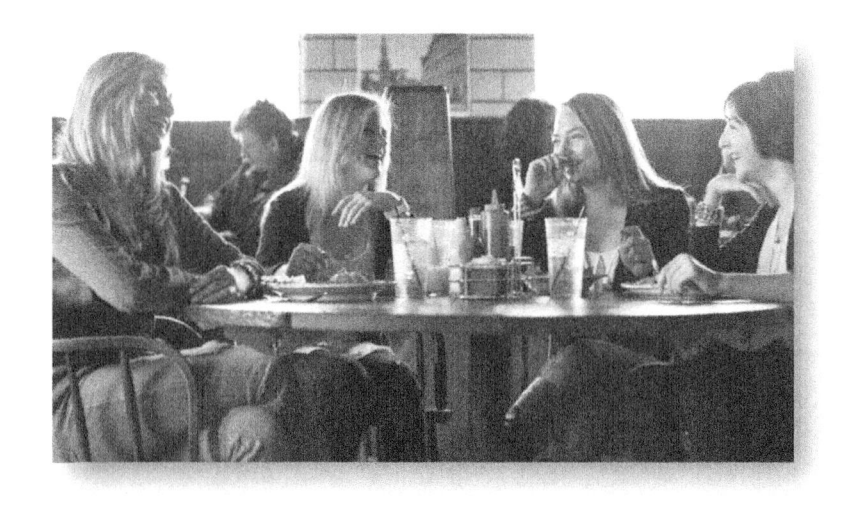

7.2 How to have a balanced food platter?

The concept of a balanced food platter is an important one when it comes to nutrition and wellbeing. A balanced food platter is one that provides our bodies with all the essential vitamins, minerals, proteins, carbohydrates, and fats we need to stay healthy. It is essential to have a balanced diet, but it can be hard to know what to include in a balanced food platter. Here are some tips to help you create a balanced food platter that will provide your body with all the nutrients it needs.

1. **Include Protein Sources** - Proteins are essential for building and maintaining muscle mass, as well as providing energy to the body.

When creating a balanced food platter, it is important to include a variety of protein sources. Some great protein sources to include on your platter are lean meats, fish, eggs, dairy, legumes, nuts, and seeds.

2. Add Healthy Fats - Fats are necessary for many bodily functions, such as hormone production and vitamin absorption, so it is important to include healthy fats on your food platter. Healthy fats include olive oil, avocados, nuts, and nut butters.

3. Include Complex Carbohydrates - Carbohydrates provide the body with energy, so it is important to include complex carbohydrates on your platter. Complex carbohydrates include whole grains, beans, peas, and other starchy vegetables.

4. Include Fruits and Vegetables - Fruits and vegetables are packed with vitamins, minerals, and antioxidants – all of which are essential for good health. When creating your food platter, aim to include a variety of different colours of fruits and vegetables.

5. Include Dairy Products - Dairy products are a great source of calcium, protein, and other essential nutrients.

To ensure your platter is balanced, include dairy products such as milk, cheese, and yogurt.

6. Consider Whole Grains - Whole grains provide the body with important vitamins and minerals, as well as fibre. When creating your food platter, aim to include a variety of whole grains such as quinoa, oats, and brown rice.

7. Add Extras - If you have room on your platter, you can add some extras to make it more interesting. Some great additions include hummus, olives, salsa, and nuts.

Creating a balanced food platter is an important step in ensuring you are getting all the essential nutrients your body needs. Be sure to include a variety of protein sources, healthy fats, complex carbohydrates, fruits and vegetables, dairy products, and whole grains. You can also add in some extras to make your platter more interesting. With these tips, you can create a balanced food platter that will provide your body with all the nutrition it needs.

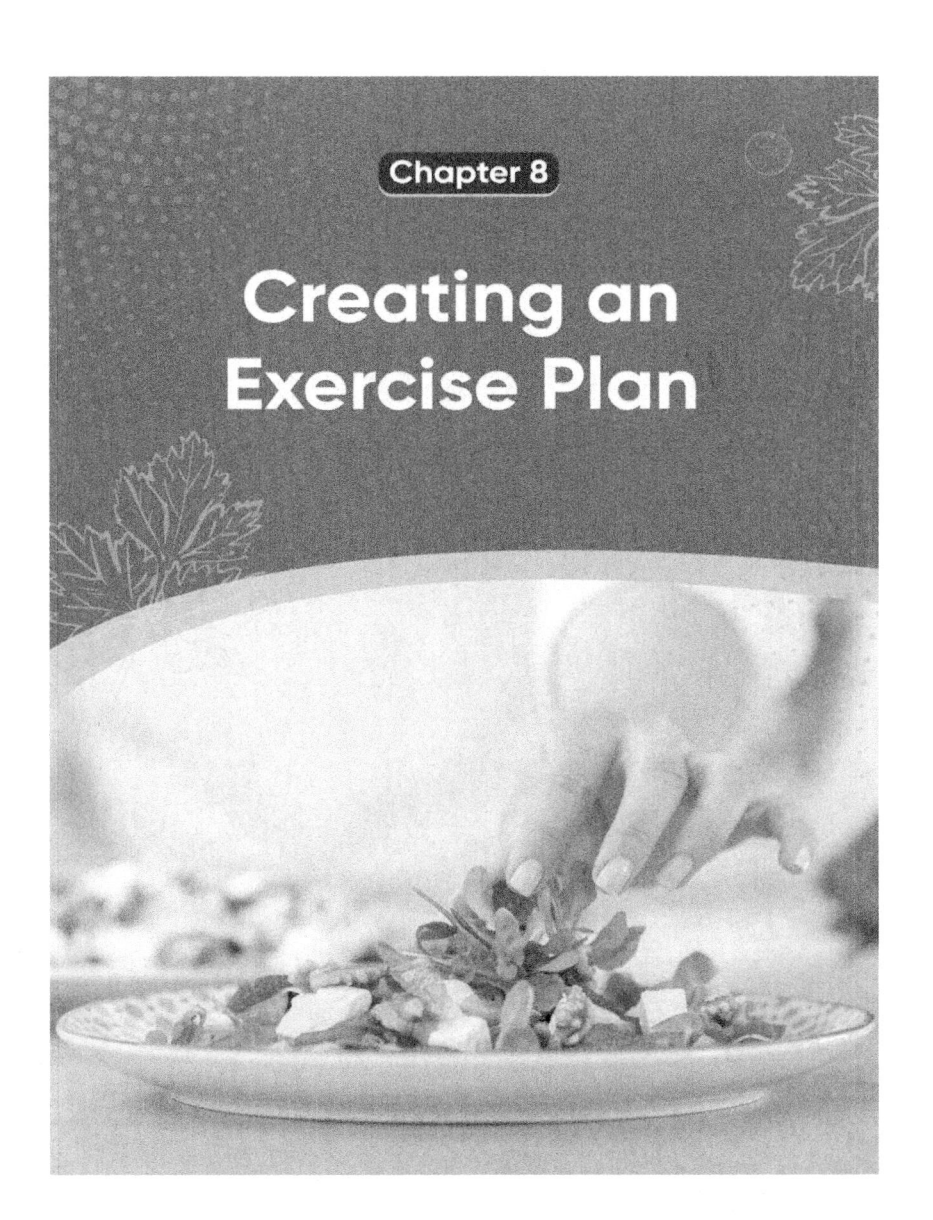

Chapter 8
Creating an Exercise Plan

Creating an effective exercise plan is an important part of achieving your fitness goals. It provides structure, allowing you to focus on specific activities that will help you reach your desired outcome. A well-designed plan should include a combination of aerobic, resistance and flexibility exercises, as well as adequate rest and recovery. By taking the time to create an exercise plan that is tailored to your individual needs and goals, you can maximize your results and stay motivated.

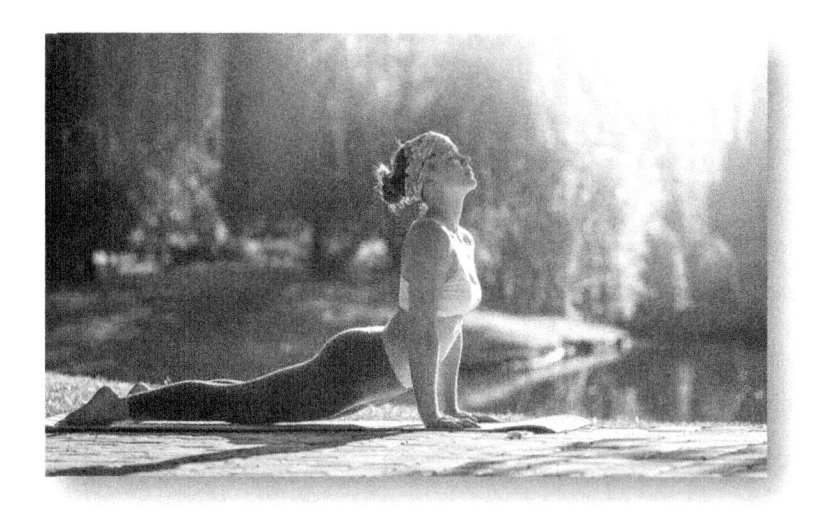

8.1 What are the benefits of exercising regularly?

Exercising regularly can be one of the most beneficial activities that you can engage in for your overall health and well-being.

Regular physical activity can help you maintain a healthy weight, reduce your risk for chronic diseases, and even improve your mental health. Here are some of the many benefits of exercising regularly.

Improved Physical Health: Regular exercise can help you maintain a healthy weight, reduce your risk of developing certain chronic diseases, and even improve your physical fitness. It can also help you to lower your cholesterol levels, reduce your risk of heart disease, and improve your overall physical health. Exercise can also increase your energy levels and help you to stay alert and focused.

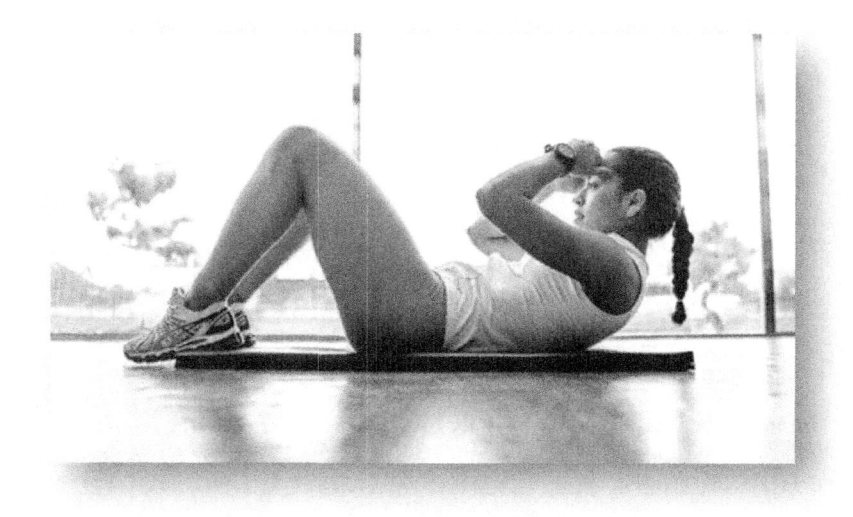

Mental Health Benefits: Regular exercise can help to reduce stress and anxiety and improve your overall mood. It can also help to improve your sleep, boost your self-esteem, and even reduce the symptoms of depression. Exercise can also help to increase your focus and concentration, making it easier to stay on task and complete tasks.

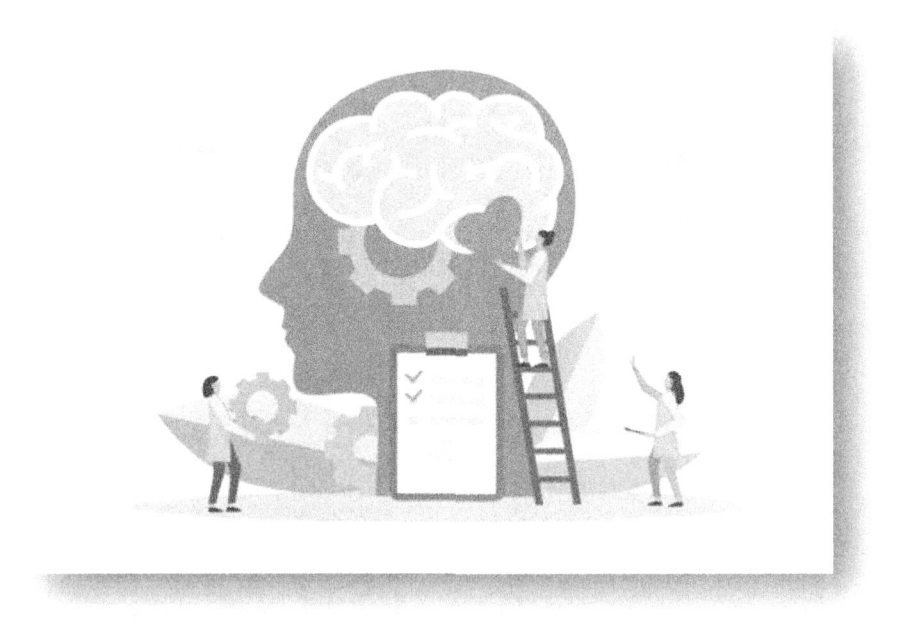

Improved Cognitive Function: Regular exercise can help to improve your cognitive function and mental performance. It can help to improve your memory, increase your problem-solving skills, and even improve your reaction time. Exercise has also been shown to help prevent age-related cognitive decline and improve overall brain health.

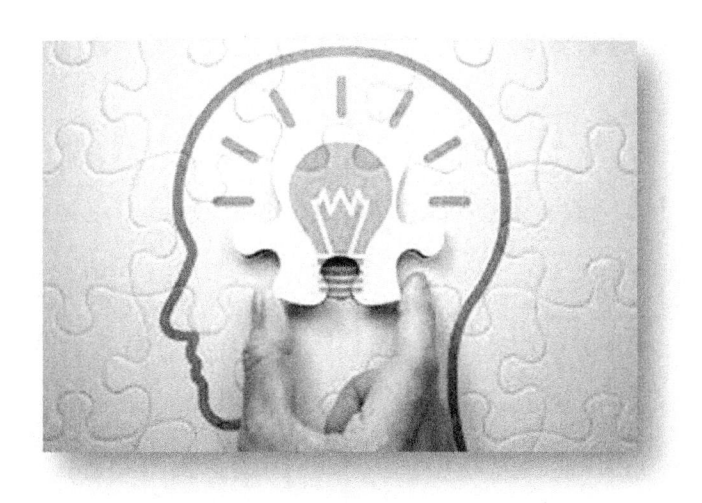

Better Quality of Life: Exercise can help to improve your overall quality of life. It can help to boost your energy levels, allowing you to do more activities that you enjoy. Exercise can also help to improve your social life, as it can provide an opportunity to connect with other people who share similar interests.

These are just a few of the many benefits that come with exercising regularly. Exercise can be an important part of any healthy lifestyle, and it can provide numerous physical and mental health benefits. So, make sure to get out there and get moving!

8.2 How to implementing an exercise routine?

A regular exercise routine is essential for maintaining a healthy lifestyle. Exercise not only keeps your body in shape, but it also helps to reduce stress and anxiety, improves your mental clarity, and increases your energy levels. When it comes to implementing an exercise routine, the key is to find a routine that works for you and to stick with it. Here are some tips for getting started.

1. Set realistic goals: Before you start your exercise routine, it's important to set realistic goals for yourself. Think about what you want to accomplish and how much time you can realistically commit to exercise.

2. Choose a type of exercise: There are many different types of exercise, from walking and running to strength training and yoga. Choose a type of exercise that you enjoy and that fits your lifestyle.

3. Find a plan: Once you've chosen a type of exercise, create a plan that includes the days and times you will exercise and the types of activities you will do.

When creating a plan, be sure to include rest days to give your body time to recover.

4. Start slow: Don't try to do too much too soon. Start with a few days of exercise per week and gradually increase the frequency as you become more comfortable.

5. Track your progress: Tracking your progress is a great way to stay motivated and keep yourself on track. Use a fitness tracking app or a journal to track how often you exercise and the type of activities you do.

6. Find an accountability partner: Find someone who will hold you accountable for your exercise routine. This could be a friend, family member, or even a personal trainer. Having someone to keep you motivated can make all the difference.

7. Have fun: Exercise should be enjoyable, so find ways to make it fun. Listen to music, watch your favorite show, or set mini-goals for yourself to keep things interesting.

Implementing an exercise routine requires dedication, but the benefits are worth it. By following these tips, you can create a routine that works for you and help you achieve your fitness goals.

Chapter 9

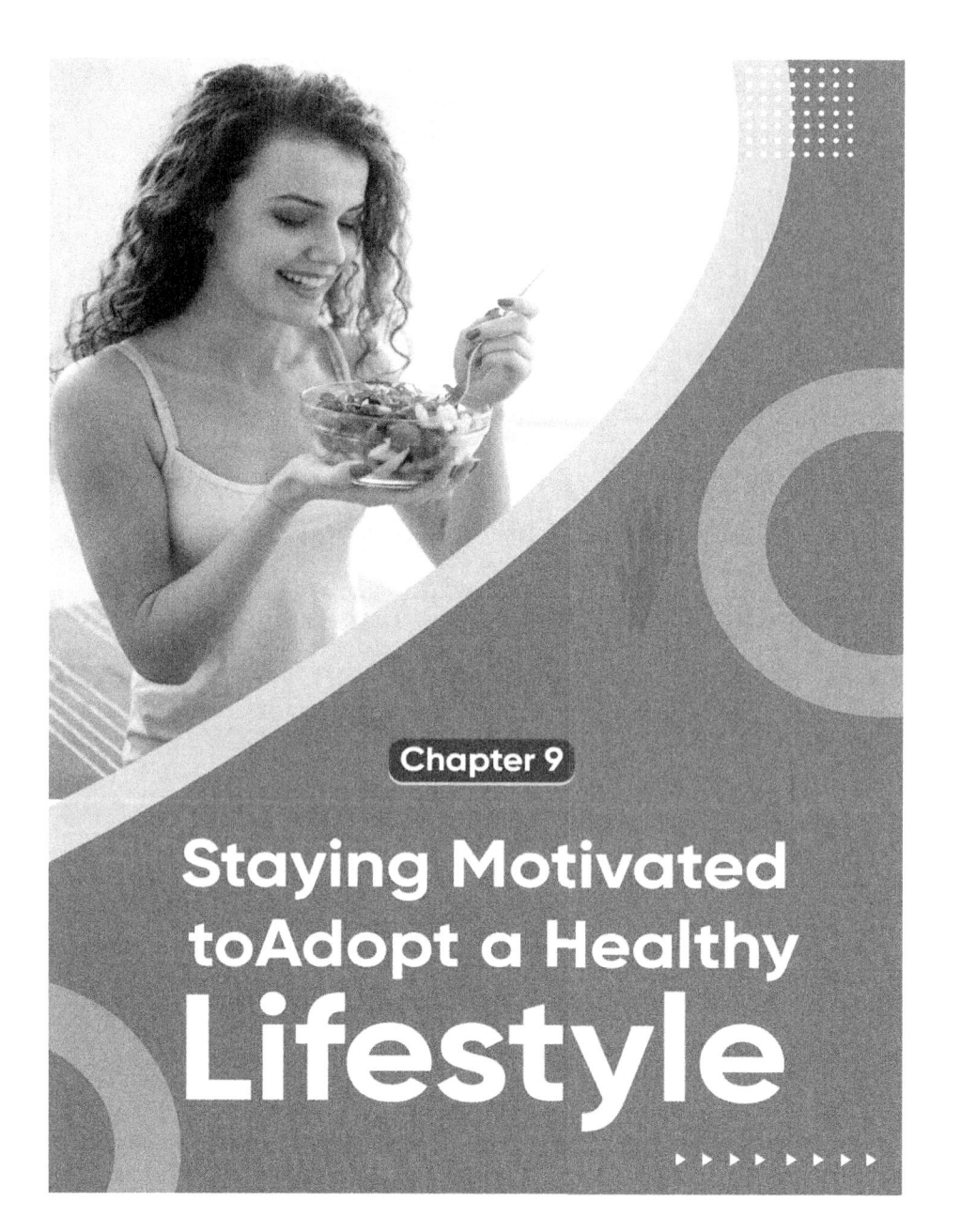

Staying Motivated to Adopt a Healthy Lifestyle

In this introduction, we will explore some of the tips and strategies that can help you stay motivated to make healthy choices and keep your body and mind in top condition.

We will also discuss the importance of staying motivated and the impact it can have on your overall wellbeing. With the right mindset and strategies, you can stay motivated to make healthy choices and achieve your health goals.

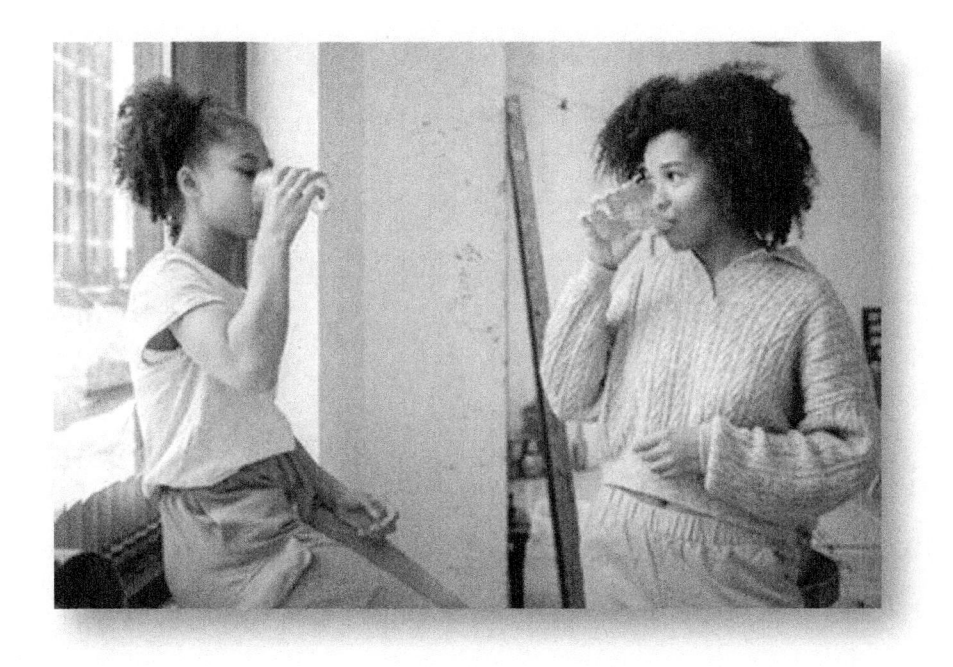

Staying motivated to adopt a healthy lifestyle can be a challenge, especially in the face of the many temptations of unhealthy habits.

However, many strategies and resources can help you stay motivated and committed to living a healthier lifestyle.

9.1 Get trained on setting realistic goals

It's essential to set goals to be successful. But just setting goals doesn't guarantee success—setting goals is only one part of a process that can lead you to success. Setting goals is crucial to planning and strategizing, executing a plan, staying motivated, and evaluating your success. This guide reviews the process for setting realistic goals and provides some example goals.

Fitness goals can be incredibly motivating, but without planning, a practical yet achievable strategy, and realistic objectives, you may end up frustrated by a lack of expected results.

When setting fitness goals, we often accidentally muddy our paths by being too desperate or too ambitious in our goal setting, but Taking a calm, confident approach to goal setting is best when setting individual goals. Think of possible small changes that you can take to achieve bigger goals.

One should always take intelligent goals can be super effective, but most people don't do it quite right.

Well, here, Smart decisions stand for something significant. It explains that you need to make a decision that's, Specific, Measurable, Achievable, Realistic, and Timely.

Process goals are focused on the actual steps it takes to reach a specific outcome rather than focusing solely on the outcome itself.

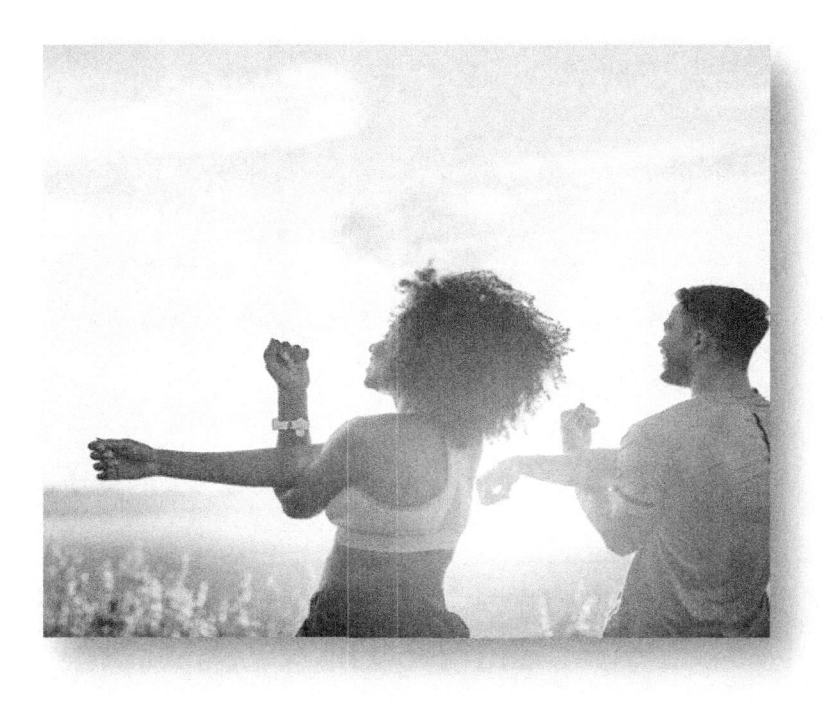

Here are some points that you can consider implementing.

Use Visualization to Find Your 'Why' - Visualizing your goals gets you started on your journey. Visualization is a popular psychological technique that can help program the mind and body to support successful goals. In fact, research suggests that visualizing yourself as successful can lead to improvements in performance, exercise frequency, focus and confidence.

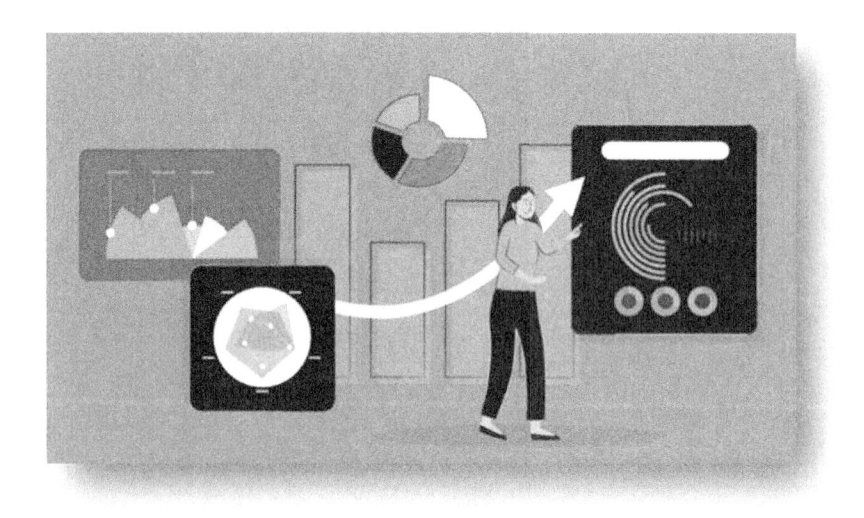

Break Big Goals Down Into Smaller Parts - Keeping your goals in sight and yourself on track to avoid a phenomenon called delayed discounting. The farther away your goal, the less the reward motivates behavior and the less dopamine your brain secretes in pursuit of that goal.

Creating set points on the way to achieving your eventual goal that keep your mind and brain on track in pursuit of that goal.

For instance, if you have a substantial weight loss goal, set your sights on achieving incremental success rather than focusing on the total weight you want to lose. Sometimes, losing 20 pounds is a great long-term goal, but it can be too long for us to wait to feel successful to focusing on one pound of weight loss at a time.

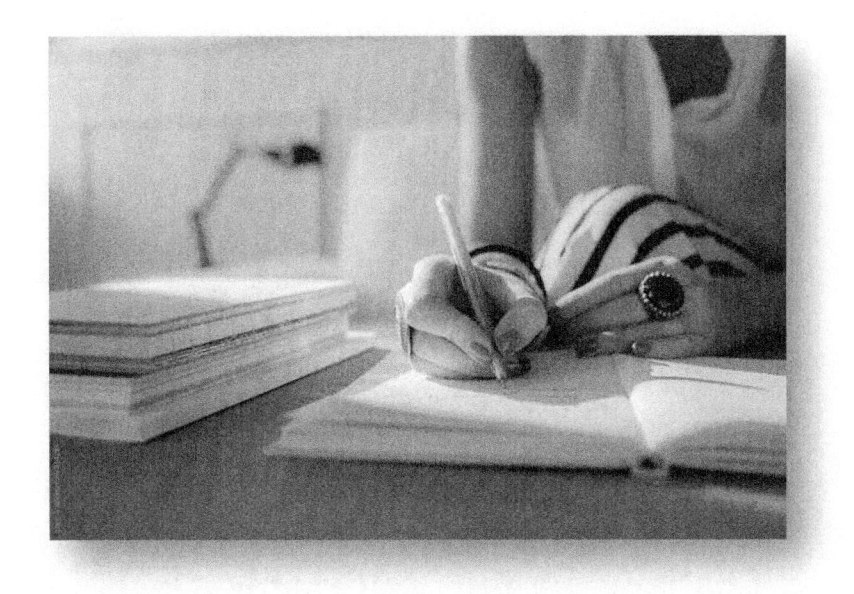

Create Daily Goal-Supporting Habits - Breaking down set points into habits, or tasks you perform each day that support your goal's success.

For instance, increasing your step count by 200 steps each day or ensuring you pack a high-protein and high-fiber snack for work each day can support an overarching training goal.

When you have clear tasks written out each day to achieve your monthly set points, it reminds you to stay focused. Practicing focus exercises can help, too. Consider deep breathing, meditation and leaving your phone idle for at least two hours a day to help you achieve your set points.

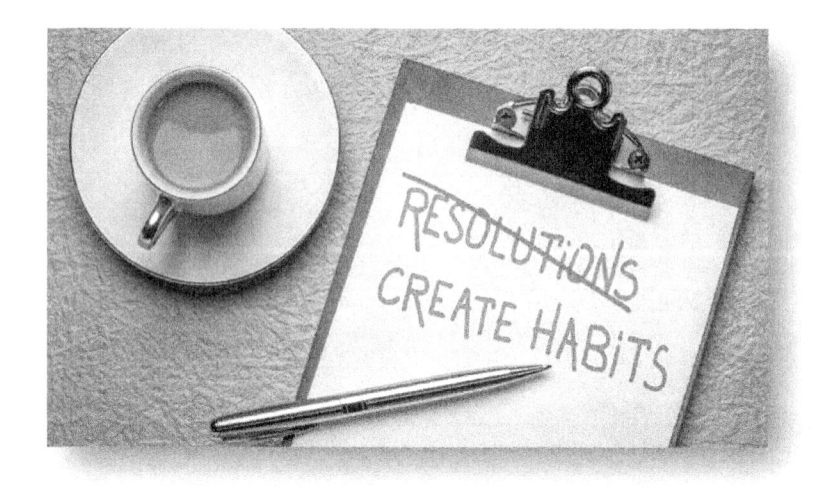

Create Challenging But Achievable Goals - One reason people don't achieve their goals is because they're either too easy or unachievable—so it's essential to find a balance when people have goals that are just barely out of reach, they're more motivated and excited to work toward them, while goals that are entirely out of reach or too easy are dismissed before they even start working toward them.

Enjoy the Process - In order to set a realistic goal, find something that interests you and brings you joy. There's no reason to train for a marathon if you hate running. Finding something you enjoy increases the likelihood of you sticking to it because you're intrinsically motivated to keep going.

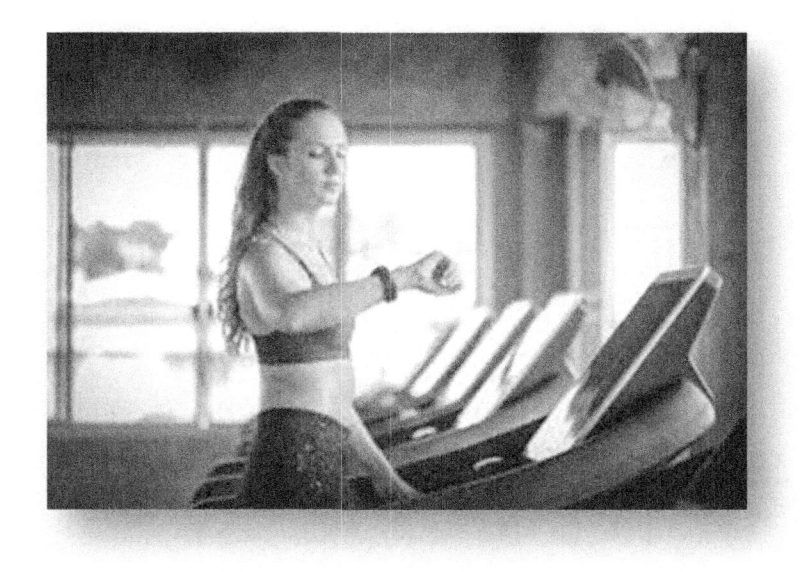

Stay Positive - Stay upbeat about hitting your goal—even if it takes longer than you'd like.

"Nothing happens overnight, no plan is perfect, and there will always be bumps in the road. Remember that your timeframe is arbitrary, and you will hit the goal at some point if you keep working for it.

Stay positive

9.2 Finding the right support system

Putting plans into action is the challenging part. Even after formulating a plan and identifying your intrinsic motivations for achieving your health goal, the tendency may be to stop there. That's why it's essential to consider the circumstances and the people surrounding you as you start your journey. After all, you are four times more likely to reach your health goals if you have a support system as you make long-term lifestyle changes.

A support system is a network of people who can give you emotional, psychological, and physical support when needed. The system can consist of friends, family, co-workers, or mentors. You can count on these people to give you a push whenever you need it and celebrate your progress with you.

Naturally, when you feel supported by the people around you to pursue your goals, you'll feel even more motivated to see them through. This is because you are not the only person invested in your progress now. Now, you have a whole support network of people who are just as eager to see you succeed in your goals.

Having a support system keeps you accountable. By informing the people around you about the goal you wish to achieve, you are inherently creating a positive form of peer pressure for yourself that pushes you to see your goal to the end.

Support can come in various forms. This support can go beyond just emotional support or simply being your motivational cheerleader. Sometimes, help can be as simple as:

- A reminder from a family member to take your medication on time.
- An offer from a friend to give you a ride to a health appointment.
- Someone is distracting you from avoiding junk food if you have resolved to eat healthier.

The support you need differs depending on the goal you have set. If your goal is professional and oriented towards work, seeking a mentor to support you and give you valuable advice would be the way to go.

A superior in your workplace or someone with experience in the field you wish to venture into would be a good choice.

Sometimes the people closest to us cannot support us and our goals or are unwilling to. In such situations, extending the circle of support a little further is a good idea by joining clubs, associations, or communities that provide an environment in which you can thrive.

With many options now available for virtual communications, your circle of support can be global.

Participating in communities of like-minded people is helpful as it allows you to communicate and receive tips from other people going through the same process and acts as a form of motivation when you see other people putting in the hours and working hard.

The Importance of Setting Healthy Boundaries.

Sometimes the people around you can be unsupportive and even downright discouraging. Words like impossible or unrealistic get thrown around, and every attempt at you trying to do better only gets met with disbelief or ridicule.

When this happens, you must establish healthy boundaries as you continue your journey. Setting healthy boundaries helps protect your self-esteem and values and, most importantly, allows you to prioritize yourself. You shouldn't let the discouraging words of others shape the way you think and act, especially if your goal will only do you good in the long run.

Just know this: support doesn't always have to be grandiose gestures or actions. Sometimes, support can be a kind word or two or even a quick text message.

What's important is showing that you care; that alone can motivate someone to reach their end goal.

9.3 How to stay motivated?

Staying motivated to achieve your goal is one of the most challenging tasks. And we are here to help you in that to stay motivated.

- Regularly review your goals and progress. Seeing progress is a great motivator in itself, and also improves your self-esteem.
- Continue to set new goals. Think about what you want to achieve next week, next month and next year. Tackle one goal at a time so you don't feel overwhelmed.
- Keep the momentum up. It takes most people about 2 months to develop a new habit, but for some people, it can take much longer. Keeping the momentum and routine helps it feel more automatic over time.
- Find mentors, for example, someone you look up to who is experienced in the habit you want to change. Finding social or support groups with the same interest can help you find a mentor.

- Surround yourself with positive people. Positive friends and family enhance your positive self-talk. This also helps to manage the symptoms of depression and anxiety.
- Use exercise as one of your daily goals to improve your mental health.

Setbacks are normal, but developing resilience can help you carry on and continue from where you left off.

Here are some tips to help you find your motivation again:

- Review your goals and see if they are realistic in the timeframe you have set. You may need to break your goal down further into smaller and more achievable goals.
- Remember why you wanted to get motivated or reach that goal in the first place.
- Take motivation from others – feel inspired by reading a book. Talk to your mentor, or friends or family who have reached similar goals to the ones you have set.
- Sometimes you just need to take a break and start afresh.

Staying motivated can be a challenge and requires dedication and hard work. To stay motivated, it is important to set achievable goals, create a plan of action, take breaks, and celebrate your successes. It is also important to surround yourself with supportive people, stay positive, and find inspiration in the things you are passionate about. Finally, it is essential to remember that it is okay to feel uninspired sometimes and to take the time to recharge and refocus on your goals.

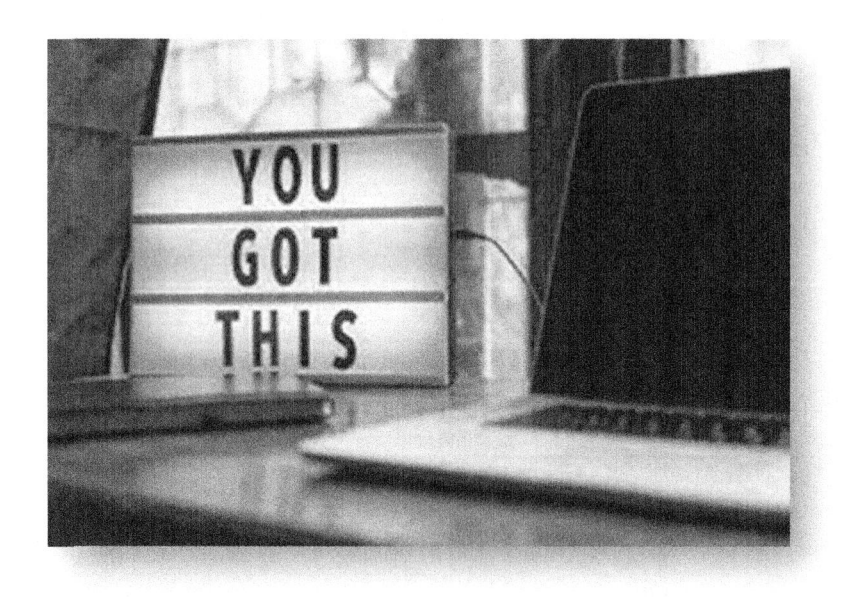

Chapter 10

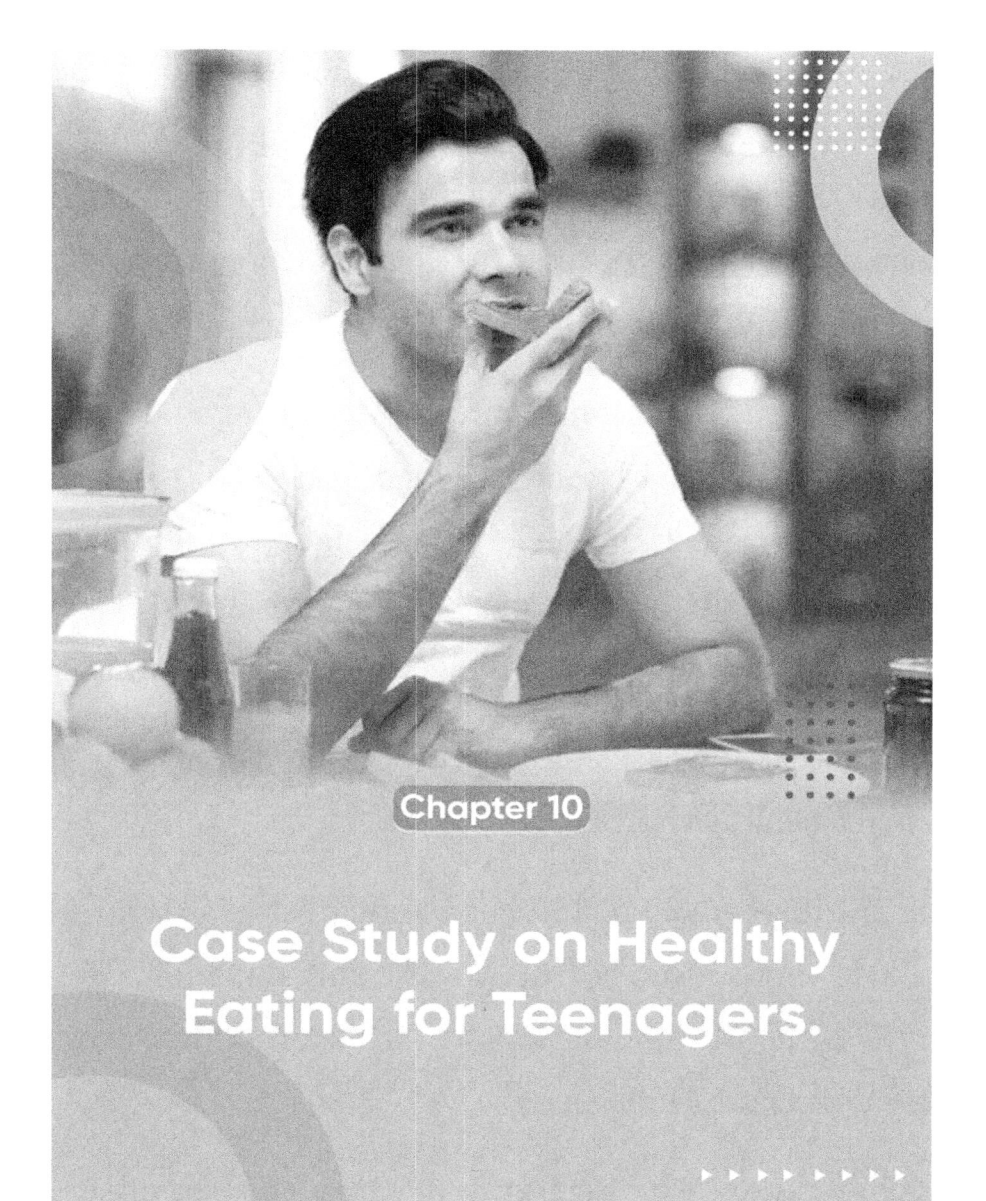

Case Study on Healthy Eating for Teenagers.

The teenage years are often a time of rapid physical growth and development, and this means that teenagers need to eat a balanced and healthy diet to support their growth and development. Unfortunately, many teenagers choose to eat unhealthy foods, such as fast food, sugar-laden snacks, and processed meals, which can lead to a variety of health problems.

The problem is that many teenagers are not eating a balanced and healthy diet, which can lead to health problems in the future. The approach is to identify the factors that influence teenage eating habits and to explore strategies that can be used to encourage healthy eating.

Well, here is the case study of a teen that can inspire you to make healthy choices.

Joe is a 16-year-old high school student who is starting to become more aware of his health and nutrition. He is active in sports and is looking to improve his overall health and performance.

Joe has always been healthy and active. His parents have always encouraged him to eat a balanced diet, but he has recently become more interested in healthy eating.

He is trying to make better food choices and has become more aware of the nutritional value of different foods.

Joe is faced with a few challenges as he embarks on his healthy eating journey. He has a lot of temptations in his environment, including fast food and unhealthy snacks. He has difficulty managing his cravings, especially when his friends are eating junk food. He also struggles to find healthy foods that he enjoys.

Joe needs to make some changes in order to start eating healthier. First, he needs to plan ahead and make sure he has healthy snacks and meals available at all times. He should also try to limit his exposure to junk food and unhealthy snacks by avoiding them as much as possible.

Joe should also focus on eating a balanced diet that consists of a variety of foods from all the food groups. He should include plenty of fruits and vegetables, lean proteins, and whole grains in his diet. He should also make sure to drink plenty of water and limit his intake of sugary drinks.

Joe is off to a great start on his journey to healthy eating. With the right planning and dedication, he can make healthy eating a part of his lifestyle. He will soon find that eating healthy can be both enjoyable and beneficial to his overall health.

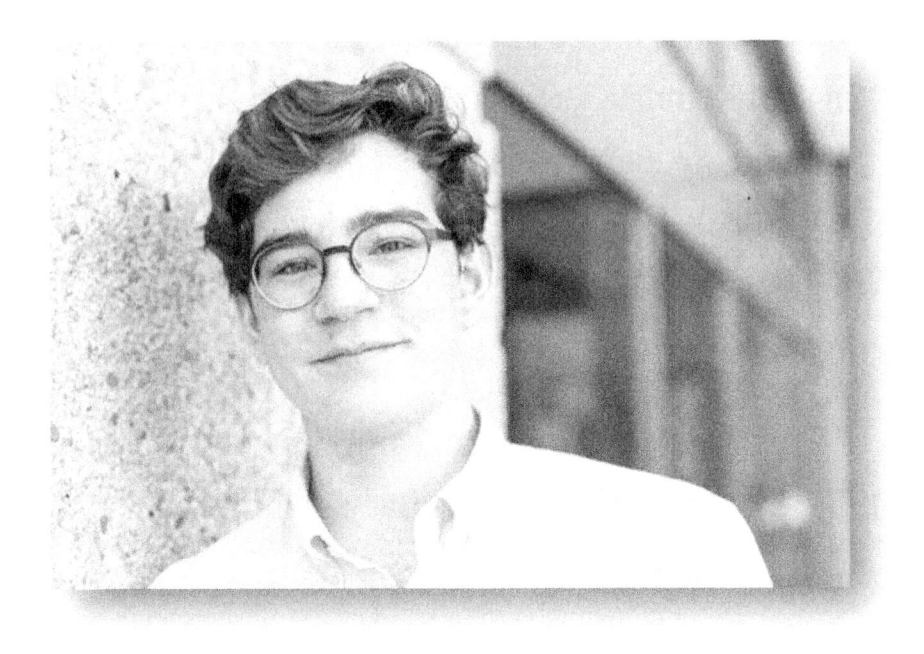

Conclusion

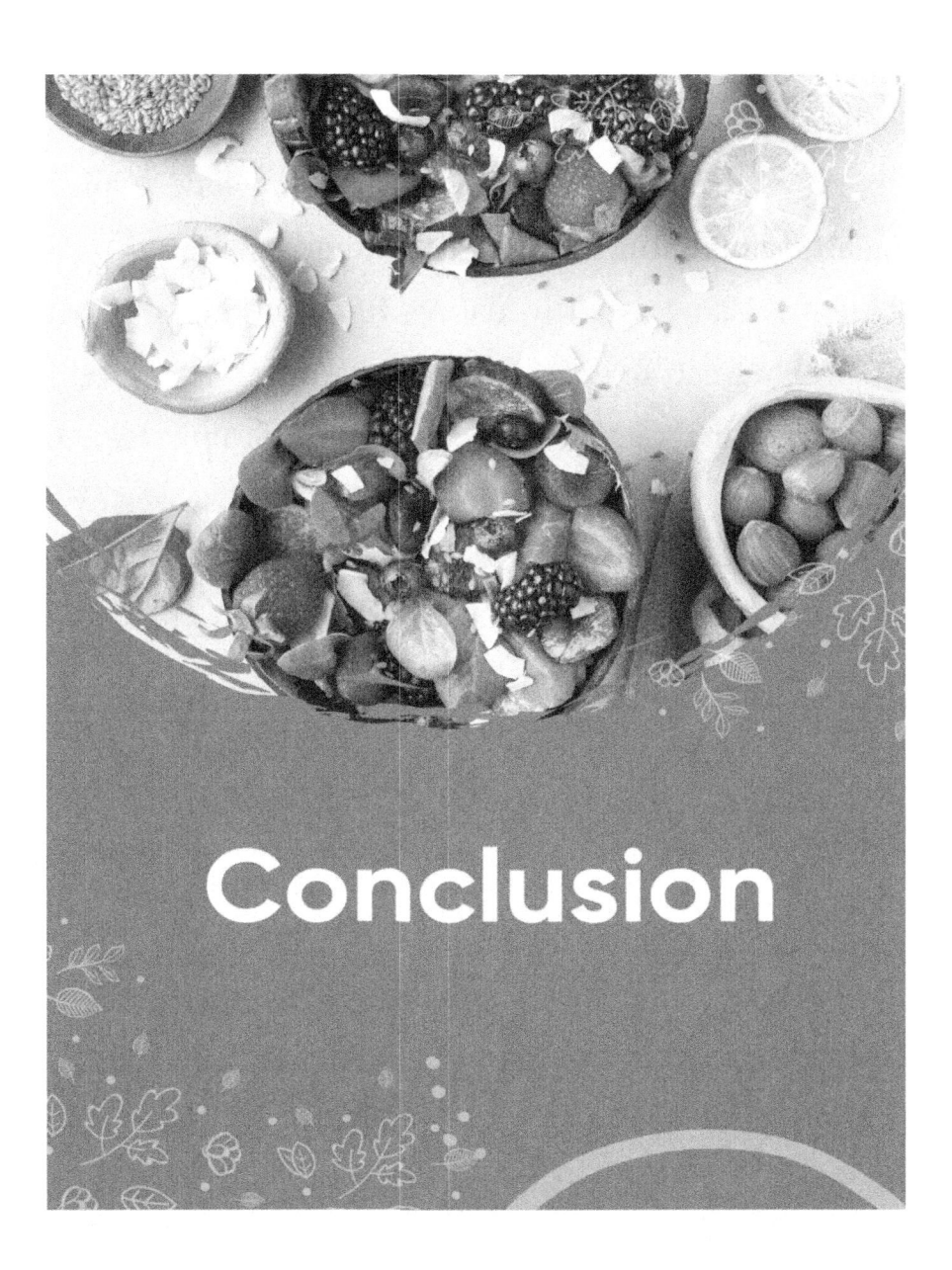

Teenagers have the potential to lead healthy and active lifestyles. Eating a balanced diet with plenty of fruits and vegetables, lean proteins, and complex carbohydrates can help them meet their nutritional needs while avoiding unhealthy foods that can lead to weight gain and health problems. Using healthy eating habits, combined with regular physical activity, can help teenagers maintain a healthy weight, build strong bones and muscles, and reduce their risk of developing chronic diseases. With proper guidance and support from their families and health care providers, teenagers can enjoy the benefits of healthy eating for a lifetime with right guidance.

Printed in Great Britain
by Amazon